BEDSIL

An Introduction

Bedside Nursing

AN INTRODUCTION

JOAN DARWIN
Director of Nursing Education
Kingston and Richmond Area Health Authority

JOAN MARKHAM
Area Nursing Officer
Kingston and Richmond Area Health Authority

BRYSSON WHYTE
Director of Nursing Education
Thomas Guy School of Nursing

THIRD EDITION

WILLIAM HEINEMANN MEDICAL BOOKS LTD
LONDON

First Published 1964
Reprinted 1966
Second Edition 1967
Reprinted 1968
Reprinted 1969
Reprinted 1970
Third Edition 1972
Revised Reprint 1976
Reprinted 1978

ISBN 0 433 07133 8

Printed in Great Britain by
WILLMER BROTHERS LIMITED, BIRKENHEAD

PREFACE TO THE FIRST EDITION

People fall ill and come into hospital for many reasons. A woman faces an operation for cancer. A man leaves home for his daily work, and an hour later arrives, bewildered, in a fracture ward with a broken leg. A child finds himself in a strange cot, parted from his family.

Some of these patients will need treatment of a highly skilled and technical kind from trained staff and senior nurses at times. All of them, however, depend on junior students and pupils and assistants for help and care and comfort throughout the day and night.

This book will describe how this care and comfort may be given, and what are the special needs of certain groups of sick people in hospital. Everyone who starts nursing wants to help people, and this book suggests how thoughtfulness and understanding as well as compassion can be of service in the daily care of the sick.

October 1964
J. D.
J. M.
B. W.

PREFACE TO THE THIRD EDITION

The third edition contains some further alterations to the original text. There is one new chapter on Community Care and several others have been extensively revised. It is hoped that the changes will help all nurses to appreciate that bedside nursing is not confined to the hospital.

October 1971
J. D.
J. M.
B. W.

ACKNOWLEDGEMENTS

The authors wish to express their thanks to Miss Winifred E. Hector for her support and encouragement in the writing of this book; to Mrs Besterman for her illustrations, and to Mr Owen R. Evans of William Heinemann Medical Books Ltd. for his guidance and cooperation.

CONTENTS

CHAPTER 1

THE NURSE IN HOSPITAL

Young women take up nursing for all sorts of reasons, some because they have wanted to be nurses since they were little girls, others because their parents have wanted them to be. Some are sure they have chosen the right career, others are beset by doubts. Some have only vague general ideas about wanting to help people, others have definite plans. One girl wants to travel round the world, another to be a health visitor, a third is going to be a mission nurse, a fourth wants to be a Nurse Tutor; these careers and many others can follow State Registration. Most girls plan to marry and raise a family at some point in their career and many will return to nursing when their children are grown up. However, for whatever reason Mary Smith takes up nursing, as soon as she puts on her uniform for the first time she will find she has become a different person; Miss Mary Smith and Nurse Mary Smith can never be the same. Nurses, like policemen, have a public image quite irrespective of their personal qualities. Over the past century the image of the nurse has changed from that of Mrs Sairy Gamp to that of the well-trained ward sister, but this is only because thousands of nurses have worked to maintain high standards of professional behaviour. Every new nurse inherits the public goodwill which has been built up for her over the years by her predecessors, and she in her turn will add something to the total picture of what nurses are like and how they behave.

It is at first both exciting and alarming for a young woman to find that the mere donning of a uniform dress and a white cap and apron makes her a person whose judgment is respected and whose advice is sought by other people. She finds that lay people assume that all nurses will be able to deal confidently with any situation from street accidents to emergency operations, and give advice on subjects ranging from matrimonial difficulties to the choice of baby foods. The first time a nurse enters a ward she feels very inadequate, she knows so little and so much seems to be expected of her. She feels that every patient in the ward must be aware of the pounding of her heart and the knocking of her knees. Gradually, however, a realization comes that she is not expected to know everything about nursing on her first ward and there are always more senior people to help and guide her until she in her turn becomes a trained nurse.

Provided one has common sense and a feeling of compassion, it is not difficult to look after someone who is not well. All mothers do it when their children are ill and many people accept it as something to be done from time to time.

Illness, however, varies in its severity. Those who have serious conditions which require surgical or special treatment are admitted to hospital. It follows that caring for these demands knowledge and that is what this book is about. It will try to give some guidance on the intelligent understanding of people who are ill in hospital.

On entry to a Nurse Training School, the student will find she is one of a class. This at once helps her adaptation to a new atmosphere. The number in the class varies from a dozen to eighty depending on the size of the school. All the students are new together; they learn from one another's mistakes and quickly form a group. The group remain together throughout training and sit their examinations together. They also finish together which is a sobering thought on one's first day.

The first few weeks of training are spent in the class-room. There is much to learn, all of it interesting because it is relevant to the performance of a nurse's duties. The design and function of the body are learnt because without this knowledge it is impossible to understand the consequence of disease or injury. The actual art and practice of nursing techniques is taught and knowledge of first aid is useful. Because the patient is a person with a family and a home, his illness cannot be studied and treated in isolation. His environment is of great importance as he comes from it and must return to it—his stay in hospital is only an interlude in his life. It is quite useless to advise the patient to avoid stairs if his flat is at the top of a building and the local housing list has two thousand names on it. So social conditions are important if patients are to be seen in true perspective. Many patients need further care on discharge from hospital so the nurse must be aware of the means of getting that help. The mental and emotional needs of the patient have a profound bearing on the whole situation, and these are also explained. These different subjects are therefore taught in the School to enable nurses to understand the problem of illness as a whole.

The popular phrase: 'The proper study of mankind is man' can well be altered to: 'The proper study of nursing is the patient'. This concept should influence the student throughout her career as well as her training. Most tutors talk to their students on the methods of actual study. They advise the nurse which text books to buy and how to use the Nursing Library, but in every case the knowledge must be linked with the patient. Knowledge is gained in order to meet the mental, emotional and physical needs of the patient more fully. Compassion and common sense enrich knowledge to produce a skilful and competent nurse.

Most students are not disturbed at the thought of the class-room work. They are familiar with school life and are prepared to come to grips with these interesting new subjects, but almost every student dreads the first actual contact with patients on the wards. Many new nurses see a ward for the first time when they go to work in it and naturally they are apprehensive. At first new nurses only visit the wards for a matter of two or three hours once a week, so that they gradually become accustomed to it. Everything is strange at first, but the routine is an established one and nurses quickly learn it. The new nurse is always accompanied when carrying out any task and it is some time before she is left to work alone. Learning and adaptation are accomplished together and in a surprisingly short space of time the nurse will find the wards a familiar place.

Nearly all potential nurses have realised that they have much to learn about patients but they do not realize how much they are in contact with other people. A hospital employs a large number of people other than nurses and doctors. Physiotherapists, radiographers, medical social workers and occupational therapists all have direct contact with the patients. Secretaries, clerks, orderlies, porters and domestic workers all have duties essential for the running of the hospital. A large staff in the kitchen deals with the food of patients and staff. Every hospital has a vast quantity of dirty linen and this has to be dealt with; sometimes the laundry is within the hospital, whilst in other places it is outside.

A highly-trained staff works in the Biochemical and Pathological Laboratories. In many of the larger hospitals there are other specialised departments all managed by skilled personnel. With some of these people the nurse has daily contact, others she may not see for months at a time. All of them are colleagues and must be treated as such, kindness and courtesy forming the basis of behaviour.

From the day she first enters the wards the nurse is in close contact with her patient. Her own appearance and personality are most important and every detail is noticed.

It perhaps seems unnecessary to emphasise that nurses must always be clean and well groomed. The majority of young nurses are this anyway but there is still a surprising amount of inattention to body odour. Deodorants must be used properly and regularly. Young people may smoke as much as they wish but it is the sick person who is easily nauseated by the smell of stale cigarette smoke which clings to all heavy smokers. Advertisements remind us that bad breath, or halitosis, is unpleasant in any situation. It is far worse when the patient is feeling ill, and nurses should be careful not to offend in this way. Perfume is also out of place at the bedside and should not be used on duty.

A young nurse who is spotless and well groomed in immaculate uniform is a most attractive sight. Nurse feels at her best and patients respond to her appearance. Physical hygiene is a great asset, but equally important is the mental and emotional stability of the nurse. Nurses quickly find that on duty in the wards they are members of a team and they have to establish relationships with their colleagues. The care of patients is founded on discipline and as nurses learn more they both see and accept the necessity for this. It is not easy for the junior nurse to appreciate the total situation and she may feel resentful when orders are given without explanation. There is not always time to explain 'the reason why' until after the event and junior nurses have to accept this fact.

Another set of relationships is established between nurses and their patients. During illness patients tend to revert to the pattern of their childhood. If this has been a happy one then the situation is quite straightforward; the patient depends on the nurse just as he depended on his mother and as he recovers so he regains his independence. But if the patient's childhood was unsatisfactory or unhappy the nurse finds herself unwittingly

in a more difficult situation which she may not at first understand. The patient's behaviour in the present is related to the
events in his past. Nurses know that all patients are treated
with kindness and patience; they grow to realize that some
need tact and wisdom as well.

There is much for a nurse to learn, but she will find it all both
interesting and absorbing. It should not be allowed to swamp
her energies, however. Nurses should cultivate interests outside
the hospital so that they find enjoyment beyond their daily
routine as well as satisfaction within it.

FURTHER READING

Barnes, *People in Hospital*. Macmillan.
Bird, B., *Talking with Patients*. Lippincott.
Burr, Joan, *Nursing of Psychiatric patients*. Ballière Tyndall and
    Cassell.
Burton, Genevieve, *Nurse and Patient*. Tavistock.
Dickens, C., *Martin Chuzzlewit*.
Gillis, Lynn, *Human Behaviour in Illness*. Faber.
Gliddon and Powell, *Called to Serve*. Hodder & Stoughton.
Nightingale, F. (1859) *Notes on Nursing*. Duckworth.
Ethics for Nurses. Nursing Times Reprint.

CHAPTER 2

COMMUNITY CARE

Good health is something which the majority of people take for granted; it is only when they are actually ill that they wonder if anything is done to prevent disease or disability. Fortunately for the community, a great deal of preventive medicine is practised, and many people spend their professional lives trying to keep the population in a state of positive health. Nurses should be aware of this work so that they can encourage people to take full advantage of the services offered.

The start of life

The foundations of good health are laid when the embryo is in the uterus. The mother should welcome the pregnancy and be physically, emotionally and mentally prepared to care for her baby when it is born. Family planning clinics help to achieve this ideal by giving advice on contraception, and help with sexual problems, so that every baby may be a wanted baby.

Once the pregnancy has started, the mother attends the antenatal clinic, where her health is checked and supervised. The growth of the foetus is assessed and its position in the uterus determined. Any deviation from normal on the part of either the mother or her baby is immediately noted, and steps are taken to deal with the situation.

Relaxation classes are conducted at the antenatal clinic; these help the mother to prepare for her labour and delivery. Both parents are encouraged to attend parentcraft classes so that they can look forward together to caring for their baby.

The Baby

The mother may have the baby at home, although the majority of births take place in hospital. In some cases the mother may be an in-patient for several days, whilst in others she may be in hospital only for the actual labour and delivery. In all circumstances the newly born baby is carefully examined and his general condition assessed to exclude the possibility of disease—this is sometimes called screening. If a congenital defect or deformity is found, the baby is immediately referred for expert advice and attention. The earlier the treatment can be started the greater the chances of either cure or alleviation of symptoms.

Whilst some congenital defects are obvious, others are obscure and only revealed on investigation. One such defect is a condition called phenylketonuria; in this there is an error of protein metabolism which has an adverse effect on the baby's mental development. Babies are screened for this abnormality by having a blood test on about the 6th day of life. The midwife takes a spot of blood from a heel prick and sends it to the laboratory for examination. If the abnormality is found, a special diet, excluding the particular protein which the baby cannot metabolise properly, is given, and the child will then develop normally.

A midwife cares for the health of the mother and her baby during the first ten days of life. After that the health visitor assumes a supervisory role for the baby and his family.

As the name suggests, the health visitor sees the family in their home surroundings. She is able to assess the social conditions and appreciate the various factors which influence the total health of the whole family. Her first care is for the new baby; her initial visit is concerned with his health and general condition. From her professional experience and background she is able to offer the mother help and advice regarding the baby's care and general routine. She invites the mother to the local child health clinic and gives her an appointment for the baby to be seen there.

At the clinic the baby is examined by the doctor and a record is made of his condition. If any abnormality is seen or suspected, or if there was any circumstance in the mother's pregnancy or labour which might affect the baby's progress, then the baby is put on a special register. The function of this register is to alert everyone so that the child's progress can be closely supervised.

The child health clinics and the health visitors are concerned with the progress of the well child; if the child is ill it is referred to his own doctor or a hospital for treatment.

When the baby is a few weeks old, the parents are asked if

H. 63

FOR INFORMATION OF DOCTOR

Tetanus

Tetanus antitoxin or booster dose of tetanus toxoid	
Subsequent injections of tetanus toxoid	

Allergies, etc.

History of Eczema	
Penicillin Sensitivity	
Other sensitivity or allergy	

DARHAMWHYTE AREA HEALTH AUTHORITY

Health Service

IMMUNISATION RECORD OF

Name _____

born on _____ /. _____ / _____

Address (1) _____

Subsequent Addresses:

(2) _____

(3) _____

(4) _____

(1500)

DARHAMWHYTE AREA HEALTH AUTHORITY

The following Immunisations are recommended

The child should be taken to _____ for the next dose on the date shown below :

ABOUT AGE *	IMMUNISATION AGAINST	DATE	TIME	DOSE GIVEN DATE	INITIALS OF DOCTOR
4 - 6 months	Diphtheria-Tetanus-Whooping Cough-Poliomyelitis (oral)				
6 - 8 months	Diphtheria-Tetanus-Whooping Cough-Poliomyelitis (oral)				
12 - 14 months	Diphtheria-Tetanus-Whooping Cough-Poliomyelitis (oral)				
15 months	Measles				
5 years	Diphtheria-Tetanus-Poliomyelitis (oral)				
5 years					
Pre-School Entry	Diphtheria-Tetanus-Poliomyelitis (Booster)				

* The ages given here are a rough guide only and vaccine may have to be given at times other than those shown on this time table. Parents should discuss the programme with family or clinic doctors.

NOTE.- Please preserve this card carefully and take it when attending as indicated above. It should also be produced to doctor or hospital if child suffers any injury.

P.T.O.

Immunisation Record Card (double-sided)

they will have him immunised, and in the majority of cases they agree. The actual immunisation may be done by the family doctor or at the local clinic. Injections of triple vaccine protect the baby against diphtheria, whooping cough, and tetanus; polio vaccine is given by mouth, and measles vaccine is given separately. The initial immunisation programme is spread over several months and booster doses are given before the child starts school. Immunisation programmes are changed from time to time.

The Pre-School Child

As the child grows his physical progress is recorded both at his visits to the clinic and by the health visitor when she sees him at home. The health visitor appreciates the need for mental stimulation and emotional security, both of which are essential for normal growth and development. Social conditions and the environment are also important, and much work is done to bring about improvements in these. This work is not spectacular, but it is important and has resulted in a better standard of child health.

The School Child

At the age of five the child must go to school, although in fact many children have been attending nursery classes for several months before the statutory age for compulsory education. The child's health record is transferred from the clinic to the school, and for the next 12 years his health and progress is recorded by the school doctor and nurse. As in the pre-school years, the emphasis is on recording normal progress, but any abnormal sign or symptom is recognised and treated without delay. Children who already have some defect or abnormality may not be able to benefit from the usual educational programme. Special schools are therefore provided, with facilities to overcome the particular handicap, e.g. schools for the deaf, the blind, or the educationally subnormal.

Immunisation against rubella is offered to schoolgirls before they reach child bearing age.

B

Young People

When young people leave school, the majority of them go straight out to work. Many firms, and some hospitals, have excellent occupational health services for their employees, and every effort is made to prevent ill health and accidents arising from conditions of employment. Health education is also practised by example as well as precept, and there are often first class facilities for sport and recreation. All these help to keep people in a state of positive good health.

The young people who go to university or college of further education find that in many cases there is a health service available to them. This service is involved with such problems as the difficulties of living away from home, drug taking, sexual problems, venereal disease. These problems are not confined to students, but many young people need help and advice when confronted with them for the first time.

Adults

In our society, adults have freedom of choice in the habits they adopt. People can choose, for instance, to smoke, or drink, or eat too much; all these habits may result in ill health. Those who smoke to excess are more likely to develop cancer of the lung, or bronchitis; obesity reduces the expectation of life and increases the tendency to heart disease, whilst those who drink or take drugs may become addicted to them. Nurses care for many patients whose illness is a direct or indirect result of their own way of life, and they should recognise that fact. A nurse who is caring for someone who is dying from lung cancer should appreciate that her own smoking habits may lead to the same end; cause and effect applies to all. Every effort should be made to present the true facts to the general public, and to help those who have a genuine desire to alter their habits. Such organisations as Weight Watchers, and Alcoholics Anonymous are of tremendous value and the churches play a big part in the rehabilitation of those who have become addicted to drugs or such social evils as compulsive gambling.

Both central and local government authorities spend time and money on health education, doing all they can to encourage people to live wisely and in safety. Some people are influenced by this publicity and their health improves in consequence; others disregard it and place their health, and sometimes their lives, in jeopardy.

The Elderly

The majority of people are in full time employment until they reach a certain age, usually between 55 and 65, when they retire. Most look forward to this, and picture themselves enjoying every minute of their leisure. The reality may be quite different unless there has been preparation for the situation beforehand. Some firms and many local authorities run courses for those contemplating retirement and there are some helpful books on the subject. Leisure must be planned for and organised if people are to enjoy it fully.

As people grow older their physical powers tend to decline but in many cases actual disability can be prevented by early diagnosis and treatment. A tentative start has been made in some areas to establish clinics for old people, where they can come for examination and advice. It is hoped that this service will expand so that eventually there will be clinics in all localities.

Many old people lose their mobility because they cannot attend to their own feet; overgrown toe nails, corns and bunions make walking difficult or impossible. A chiropody service is therefore invaluable and many Health authorities provide one.

An adequate diet is essential if people are to remain fit and well. Old people may not find it easy to obtain this, either because of the expense, or because of the difficulties of shopping, preparing or cooking food. Luncheon clubs enable the elderly to have one good meal a day at a very reasonable cost and at the club they meet their own contemporaries. Day Centres have more extensive facilities than Luncheon Clubs and as the name implies, the elderly spend the day there. They are collected from their homes in the morning and returned to them in the late afternoon. Many day centres have facilities for bathing and hairdressing and the chiropodist may hold his clinic there. There may be handcraft classes, talks, social gatherings and entertainments, and of course, meals are provided.

For those who are unable to leave home there are many health and welfare services, although the demand for these exceeds the supply. The 'Meals on Wheels' service provides midday meals; home helps go into the home to clean, cook, wash, or do the shopping; an incontinent laundry service takes bed and personal laundry from those who are incontinent; incontinent pads are supplied to those who need them, and various nursing aids and appliances are loaned out when necessary. The home nurse and the home bather visit those who are ill or incapacitated and in many areas there is a night sitting service to provide help at night.

It is not only the elderly who require health and welfare services; a large number of younger people are disabled in some way and the services attempt to cover their needs. The service provided by the community is supplemented by an enormous amount of voluntary work and many nurses will already have had personal experience of this through their membership of a society such as the British Red Cross Society or the St John Ambulance Brigade. As the demand and need for the services grows so the role of the volunteer becomes more important and nurses should recognise the value of their contribution.

This chapter has presented a brief outline of the available preventive and supportive health services, but it should be appreciated that these alter as social and medical conditions change. Every decade brings its own problems and fresh services are created to meet new demands. In every case, however, the services cost money and need skilled people to run them. Any authority could provide a comprehensive service if it were given an unlimited supply of money and personnel. As this Utopian state of affairs will never be attained, each area health authority has to do its best within a limited framework, using its resources to give the best service it can.

FURTHER READING

You; Your Health; Your Community. Leff. Wm Heinemann Med. Books.

Chisholm, M. K. *An Insight into Health Visiting.* Ballière Tindall & Cassell.

CHAPTER 3

THE PATIENT'S ENVIRONMENT

Hospitals are meant to serve the needs of the people living in a particular area. These needs may change considerably over the years as the differences in the patterns of living affect patterns of disease. Although the changes may be dramatic, such as those brought about by the discovery of penicillin, they may be so gradual that people living at the time never notice the beginning of a new trend, but the hospital reflects them faithfully as it adapts itself to the new demands. The ward that held diphtheria patients in 1880 may have been turned into a gastro-enteritis unit in 1930 and in 1974 be a chest surgery unit for patients with carcinoma of the lung. The study of graphs of the incidence of disease shows that some, like plague, have gone altogether, but others have been 'replaced' by different conditions. Almost as many children now die in road accidents as used to die of diphtheria and more people died in London from the effects of the 'smog' of 1952 than from a cholera epidemic in the 1860's.

Many factors are responsible for the type of illness a patient has, some of which are known and understood and some not. There are causes arising within the patient himself and those affecting him from without. Some conditions, such as haemophilia, are due solely to hereditary factors which are passed on from one generation to the next in the genes. There is as yet very little that can be done to prevent or influence the occurrence of such diseases. Other conditions result almost entirely from external causes, falling and breaking a leg for example. Today, doctors recognize more and more that many illnesses arise as a result of a combination of factors. Sadness as well as staphylococci may predispose to boils.

HISTORICAL FACTORS

Among the forces influencing the pattern of disease is the age in which the patient lives. Study of the bills of mortality for London in 1664 shows that although patients died of 'gowt', 'grief', and 'griping in the guts', none of them was affected by

nuclear radiation. Infants were smothered (over-lain) but not
with plastic bags. People were struck by lightning but not elec-
trocuted. In the time of the first Queen Elizabeth the expectation
of life was about twenty-four years, in the time of Queen Elizabeth II it is nearer seventy years, so that the pattern of degenerative disease has changed.

OCCUPATIONAL FACTORS

The patient's job is another factor in the causation of disease.
Studies have been carried out comparing the incidence of certain
conditions in groups of workers doing different jobs. All sorts
of fascinating facts emerge. Why should leather workers be so
high on the list of those likely to develop peptic ulcers? Why do
miners suffer more from rheumatism than farm workers? Why
should 'women overlookers' have a neurosis rate three times
that of foremen? It is very difficult to disentangle cause from
effect. Does it mean that people of a certain type are good at,
or tend to choose, a particular job, or has the job itself some
associated strain or risk attached to it? Both can be true; square
pegs can become ill through trying to fit round holes and some
jobs do have special health hazards connected with them.
Workers in dusty trades for example may, unless protected,
develop lung conditions from the constant inhalation of certain
types of dust. Coal miners may get a condition called silicosis
from the inhalation of minute particles of silica; asbestos miners
may contract a similar condition from asbestos dust, and oxy-
acetylene welders may damage their eyesight unless they wear
goggles. People who work with machinery, unless it is correctly
guarded, are obviously more likely to have 'accidents with
machinery' than those who work at other jobs. Even nurses, if
they were not safely protected by B.C.G., could be said to run a
special risk through the possibility of their exposure to tuber-
culous infection. In most instances all these special risks are
known, and workers in such jobs are protected by Acts of
Parliament, such as the Factory Acts, which lay down, among
other things, the standards of safety for those working in potentially hazardous jobs. Indeed, if it can be proved that in spite of
precautions, the patient's job has directly contributed to his
illness, there may be special pensions and other forms of compensation available to him.

EMOTIONAL FACTORS

This does not explain why, when two people are doing the same job, one should become ill and the other not. There is another factor which cannot be disregarded, and that is the emotional makeup of the individual. For example, people who are anxious and worried often tend to develop illness more readily than those who take life more calmly. It is sometimes difficult to believe this, or to accept that illness has any but a physical cause. However, people can accept that the emotion of grief is accompanied by the physical manifestation of a flow of salt water from two small glands below the eyebrows (tears) and that the emotion of anxiety may be accompanied by a feeling of discomfort in the bowel, or a contraction of the muscles of the bladder. It is clear therefore that there is a link between emotion and physical changes in normal life.

Many people suffer from anxiety in certain situations, such as waiting to go into an examination room; but some people live permanently in this state as if they were spending their whole life outside the door of an intangible, invisible examination room of whose very existence they were unaware. As a result of this prolonged anxiety physical changes may occur.

The roots of such anxieties are complex. They may arise from causes as diverse as some incident in childhood which the patient has forgotten but his nervous system has not; from the pressure of holding down a difficult job, or from an unhappy family situation. It must be remembered that the patient can no more control these bodily changes than he can control the working of his nervous system, and it is not his fault if he is more prone to certain types of disease.

BACTERIAL FACTORS

Even in the nineteenth century, illness was often due to direct infection by bacteria carried by flies or lice, or in contaminated water or milk. The resistance of the population to disease depended very largely upon whether or not they had money. Rich Victorians were comfortable, well fed and well housed. Poor Victorians lived in conditions of squalor and misery; the infant mortality rate was high, and poverty and malnutrition were responsible for many deaths. Those who learn about water and sewage systems today may think that all the pioneer work in this field is over. The figure of Dr John Snow dramatically halting the progress of a cholera epidemic by his command: 'Take the handle off the pump, had dwindled into that of an ordinary public health inspector doing a routine job in every town in England. The Victorian lady carrying soup to the poor has been replaced by the welfare services and the Department of Health and Social Security. However, some conditions still exist which could be eliminated by public health measures—notably air pollution. The comparative death rates from bronchitis in England and other countries of Europe show how serious a problem it is, and although smoke pollution is not the only cause, it is certainly a contributory factor. In fact, bronchitis could now qualify for the title of 'The English Disease', which was once held by rickets. In spite of the un-doubted association between polluted air and disease, the public pay very little attention. People who would complain if they were served with an unwrapped loaf are content to breathe their share of the tons of contaminated soot which fall on their town each day without doing anything about it. However, although public health measures affect the health and happiness of the community, the centre of life for most people is their home and family.

HOUSING FACTORS

The effect of a house on the people who live in it is not just a matter of bricks and mortar, as local authorities soon found out when they first started rehousing slum families. They moved the families without moving their way of life. Most people think of the traditional English village as a number of picturesque cottages clustered round a church, and expect there to be some sort of community spirit and feeling. It takes longer to grasp that the same spirit and feeling can be present in a few rows of mean streets clustered round a public house. It was not until people from such areas were rehoused that it was realized that sudden removal from familiar surroundings can cause home-sickness and loneliness which can seriously affect mental health. It must not be thought that the people who lived in slums were so foolish as not to want better housing. No normal woman wants to share a lavatory with two other families or carry all her water from an outside tap. But just as it is now known that a baby needs cuddling and love for its normal mental development, so it is known that a family needs friends, neighbours and familiar surroundings for its mental health. Modern architects are slowly learning these lessons and 'building-in' friendliness to new estates by their placing of back doors and kitchen windows—so that women can meet and gossip easily.

FAMILY FACTORS

The relationships of members of a family with each other and with the community have an effect on the personality of the individual. Some patterns of living are normal for one community, some for another. It is accepted that a woman when she marries takes her husband's name and goes to live in his town; that the eldest son succeeds his father, that the man is the head of the household. Other peoples think differently, and in their society the man will go to the woman's household when he marries and becomes part of her family. In some tribes it is the youngest son who succeeds his father, in others, the eldest. If in any society the pattern is reversed, it will have some effect on the members of the family. For example, if the mother were to become the sole bread-winner, because the father was out of work or unable to earn, the children might tend to think less of their father.

Children need a stable environment in their early years if they are to have normal emotional development. The first person they are usually aware of apart from themselves is their mother. This first relationship is the crucial one. If it cannot be established successfully the child can never learn to make an entirely normal relationship with anyone else. For instance, if an infant is separated from his mother (perhaps because she is ill) and no stable substitute is found, he may become withdrawn and apathetic, failing to thrive. This may occur if a child is moved through a series of foster homes. The next person with whom a child makes a relationship is his father. He admires his father whom he thinks of as a powerful protector, but hates to share his mother with his father. Once he has learnt to make these relationships with his mother and father he is ready to extend his range to all the other people he is going to meet in life. Abnormal emotional development, such as that caused by the break-up of the home at a crucial time in the child's life, can alter a whole personality and make it more likely that the person concerned will suffer from certain types of illness. It may seem a haphazard arrangement that such an important job as growing normal people is left to two such amateurs as the average mother and father, but the secret of success is love. If the child is loved and wanted, his parents can do him very little harm; it is the unwanted child who is in danger.

Thus there are many strands which make up the patient's personality and the illnesses from which he may suffer are seldom the result of a single factor. Seeing the patient wrenched from the context of his daily living when he is in hospital makes the doctor's job a very difficult one, and nurses will observe how patiently the doctor reconstructs the patient's background, because only when he has a complete picture can the treatment be really effective. No two patients are ever affected alike by a standard text book disease, and the art of nursing, for it is an art, is in learning to nurse a person, not a disease.

FURTHER READING

Dance, Meredith. *Preventive Medicine for Nurses and Social Workers*. E.U.P.

Haggard. *Devils, Drugs and Doctors*. Heinemann.

Mansfield, *Avoidable Death*. Cassell.

Newsom, John and Elizabeth, *Patterns of Infant Care in an urban community*. Pelican.

Newsom, John and Elizabeth, *Four years old in an urban community*. Pelican.

Young, *Family and Kinship in East London*. Pelican.

On the State of the Public Health. H.M.S.O.

CHAPTER 4

THE NURSE AND THE
PATIENT'S ARRIVAL

When a patient enters hospital he gives up his world of home, wife, children and job to enter another world with very different values. Nurses and doctors who work in this strange world of hospital have always to remember that it is not the real one, and although its calm certainties and secure routines relieve the patient of the dreadful weight of decision whilst he is ill, he will one day have to return to the real world and resume his responsibilities. Patients who enter hospital do so in two ways; either they are sent by their doctor to 'Out-Patients' and thence put on a waiting list, or they are admitted as an emergency following an accident or sudden illness. When he is first admitted the patient has two concerns, the situation at home, and the strange unknown world of hospital.

BACKGROUND PROBLEMS

His concerns at home may be financial, personal or social. His whole livelihood may depend upon himself if he has a one-man business, and this may be ruined if his stay in hospital is prolonged. If he works for a 'boss' his job may not be kept open for him, or even if it is waiting for him, his health insurance money may not be enough to cover his commitments and supplementary pension may be needed to supplement his income. His problem may range from the frustrating, (final examinations next week), to the tragic, (his wife very ill in another hospital), to the irritating, (he forgot to cancel the milk), to the pathetic, (he is a pensioner who lives alone and his dog is fretting for him).

Women, on admission, have a whole range of problems. The most common is worry about the children or perhaps an old person for whom they have been responsible. If there has been time to make arrangements, the children may be safely with granny, but if the admission has been rushed, other solutions must be found. These range from having a home help in the house, to sending the whole family to a residential nursery or children's home. It may be possible for father to take time off his work to look after the children or even make use of a day nursery for the younger ones if a kind neighbour will give the older ones their tea when they come home from school. Even a wife without children will worry about how her husband is managing on his own, is he eating proper meals? Has he broken all the best china? The unmarried worry about boy-friends and fiancés; are they coming to visit? Are they going off with other girls?

The following true examples illustrate this point:

Miss H., a middle-aged spinster, was seen in 'Out-Patients' in May and told that she would be admitted in 'a few months'. As she was responsible for an elderly, crippled aunt she asked if some more definite time could be arranged so that she might make arrangements for the care of her relative. She was told that she would be admitted in July. She arranged with her sister to take her holiday from work in July so that the old lady's care would be assured. July came, the sister took her holiday but no word came from the hospital. Finally, in August, Miss H. was sent for, but by this time there was no one free to look after the old lady and Miss H. was admitted in great distress, worrying about the hasty and unsatisfactory arrangements she had had to make, which in addition had proved very expensive.

Mr B., a young, single man, had a good job which was being kept open for him. His National Health Insurance money was coming in and his landlady was keeping his room for him. What worry could he have? Mr B. was a keen racing pigeon enthusiast and owned a pigeon loft and fifty birds. His main concern was these pigeons and who would feed them.

Mrs O. was a married woman with seven children, all under ten. Her main concern was with the safety of her children as she did not want to leave them with her husband who drank heavily. In addition she was worried about what her husband might do to the flat in which they lived, as he had on previous occasions sold furniture and bedding. There was another woman, and this also concerned Mrs O. who loved him and had for years held the home together and realised that all her work might be undone in the few weeks she was in hospital.

PERSONAL PROBLEMS

Apart from background worries the patient will be concerned about his illness. Could it be cancer? Will he be able to work at his old job after the operation? What is an operation like? Is it true that they sometimes start before you are asleep? What will the ward be like? Will there be any privacy? Will he have to use a bedpan? These and a thousand other questions must pass through the patient's mind as he awaits admission.

FIRST IMPRESSION

Finally the appointed day arrives and the patient and his friends present themselves at the hospital door. They are in a state of great apprehension and every word and gesture of greeting is noted. Everyone in the chain of admission, porter, receptionist, nurse and sister has an important part to play: a careless word or a thoughtless reply may colour the whole of the patient's subsequent attitude to the hospital. The patient must never suspect that the porter's rheumatism is bad, the receptionist's boyfriend has jilted her, or that he has been admitted to the ward on the morning the pipes burst. The secret of a successful admission is for every one to appear to be expecting the patient. If all admission procedures ran as smoothly as they should this would indeed be the case, but nurses must learn to deal as calmly with the unexpected patient as with the expected one. A swift glance at the admission slip before welcoming the patient by name is easily managed, and the patient feels that his individuality has been preserved. The nurse should take this opportunity of introducing herself to the patient.

TAKING PARTICULARS

If it is a routine admission the taking or checking of particulars is vital. It is obvious that the name, age and address of the patient must be recorded. Their own doctor's name and address are needed so that liaison between the hospital and the general practitioner can be maintained. The religion is noted so that the appropriate minister may be informed. The next-of-kin should be noted with extreme care, a married patient may be separated and not wish their spouse informed; nurses must use tact when eliciting such information. The importance of some means of communication with the next-of-kin cannot be too much stressed. Most people wish to be with their relatives when they are very sick or dying, thus whoever has to call the relatives must have sufficient data on which to work.

Sisters and daughters marry and change their names, no one should have to waste time asking for Miss Smith when they really want Mrs Jones. Telephone numbers are not complete unless the exchange is recorded. Nearly everyone without a telephone knows some neighbour who will take a message at night, and most employers are very accommodating about messages in the daytime if they are asked. The police are very helpful but sister will think twice before adding another task to the duties of an overworked constable. If the number given has to be that of the nearest police station, a note should be made of its address. The nurse taking particulars of this kind should imagine herself in the position of the night sister having to contact relatives in an emergency.

THE NURSE'S RESPONSIBILITIES

When admitting a patient a consent to anaesthetic and operation form must be signed if necessary. The patients identification label is checked and fastened to his wrist. Patients find this easier to accept if the reason for its use is explained first. When this and all other particulars have been checked the nurse makes her observations on the patient, including; taking the pulse, temperature and respiration, weight, blood-pressure and obtaining a first specimen of urine. It may or may not be necessary for the patient to have a bath on admission, but it is usual for him to change into pyjamas and dressing gown. His family can then take his clothes home if that is the routine of the hospital. In some cases it may be necessary to inspect the hair to make sure there is no infestation, and any 'doubtful' head can then be combed. The general state of the patient can be observed during all these formalities; is he calm and relaxed or tense and anxious? Does he appear to have any special worries?

Both he and his relatives will ask a great many questions and the nurse must answer them as freely as she can. Many hospitals have a booklet printed with information about visiting times, ward routine and other 'hints for patients' and the nurse must make sure that the patient has one. She must also ensure that the relatives have an opportunity to see sister before they leave. When the relatives have said good-bye to the patient and gone, he can be introduced to his neighbours and settled with a book or newspaper. It is helpful to tell him the time of the next meal or the possible time of the doctor's visit so that he has something to look forward to.

EMERGENCY ADMISSIONS

Emergency admissions are rather different and special preparations are made for them. The ward may admit emergencies for a definite period, or may always be geared to receive them. If patients are likely to be admitted from the street after accidents, a specially prepared bed is made ready for them. Cradles, fracture boards, extra waterproof-covered pillows are kept in readiness so that they may be inserted as required. One of the difficulties connected with emergency admissions is informing relatives; the patient, if conscious, may be very worried about them and must be reassured that they are being informed. This duty usually falls to the police, who perform it admirably, but nurses should always remember the state of extreme fear and shock caused by such news and deal gently with the relatives when they reach the hospital.

Clothing and valuables should receive special attention. A list of property should be made and checked and signed by two people. The valuables should then be stored in the hospital safe and the receipt handed to the patient or his relations.

Thus the patient enters the strange world of *hospital* and puts his life into the hands of strangers. Doctors and nurses should remember that the surrender is both voluntary and temporary and that they should respect the dignity of the patient as a fellow human being and not take advantage of being set in authority over him.

FURTHER READING

Barnes, *People in Hospital*. Macmillan.
McGhie, *The Patient's Attitude to Nursing Care*. Livingstone.
Vaizey, *Scenes from Institutional Life*. Faber.

CHAPTER 5

THE NURSE AND THE
PATIENT'S COMFORT—PERSONAL HYGIENE

THE SKIN

Probably the most familiar tissue in the whole body is the skin. Like many other familiar objects little notice is taken of it. It is washed at intervals, subjected to extremes of heat and cold and frequently torn or cut, yet everyone grumbles if it shows any sign of reaction to this harsh treatment. As it is part of the living body, the skin is composed of cells. Like all other cells, these have a span of life, and when they reach the end of this, they die, having been replaced by new cells. The new cells are replaced from the inside and the worn out ones are shed from the surface. So the skin really consists of a layer of cells, the young active ones on the inside being pushed up in turn to the middle of the layer. Desiccation starts and the cells gradually reach the surface from whence they are shed.

The skin varies in colour with the amount of pigment contained in the cells. It also varies in thickness with its situation, being thickest on the soles of the feet and palms of the hands, and thinnest on the delicate structure of the eyelids. In the deeper layers of the skin are the blood vessels which play a very important part in the regulation of body temperature. If the body needs to lose heat, these vessels dilate, and a large amount of blood flows through them. The skin becomes flushed and heat is lost from the surface by radiation. On the other hand, if the body needs to conserve its heat, the vessels are constricted and very little blood flows through them. The skin is white and cold to the touch; little heat is lost. Also connected with the regulation of temperature are the sweat glands. These are situated in the deeper layers of skin and are more numerous in certain parts of the body, e.g. armpits, forehead. The glands produce sweat which is composed of water and salts (principally sodium chloride) and evaporation of it from the skin surface helps to reduce the temperature of the body.

The skin is also a most important sense organ, conveying

c

much information about the environment to the brain. Receptor nerve endings in the skin can appreciate heat, cold, pain or pressure and this information is immediately relayed to the spinal cord and brain. Again, the distribution of these nerve endings varies with the parts of the body, the finger-tips and mouth being particularly sensitive.

Two structures, hair and nails, are peculiarly developed portions of the skin and are known as appendages. They are still living structures, a fact which is immediately obvious when one

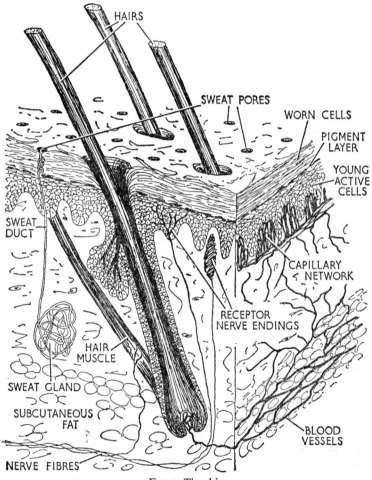

HAIRS

SWEAT PORES

WORN CELLS

PIGMENT LAYER

YOUNG ACTIVE CELLS

SWEAT DUCT

CAPILLARY NETWORK

RECEPTOR NERVE ENDINGS

HAIR MUSCLE

SWEAT GLAND

SUBCUTANEOUS FAT

BLOOD VESSELS

NERVE FIBRES

FIG. I The skin

considers the length they will reach if left uncut. Although so very different in appearance from the rest of the skin it is convenient to consider them with general care and cleanliness.

CLEANLINESS

Skin gets dirty quite quickly. In addition to the dead cells being shed from the surface and sweat glands continually producing perspiration, dust settles on the skin. Contact with dirty surfaces increases the contamination, even though clothing and gloves may be worn. If sweat is allowed to become stale it smells and this adds to discomfort. All the body surface needs to be washed though those parts which are exposed, *e.g.* hands and face, need more frequent attention. People who are ill need a daily bath just as much as people who are well and active.

Bathing in the Bathroom

Many patients are allowed to go to the bathroom to have a bath in the usual way. Nurse should see that the bathroom is warm, that the patient has all his toilet articles, soap, flannels, towels, and that the water is of the temperature to suit that particular patient. Hot and cold water should be run in simultaneously. Hot water in hospitals is often of a very high temperature and if this is run in first and then cold water is added, it is possible for the patient to step into a bath that is much too hot, although feeling the surface gives a deceptive sense of security. Some patients may need help to get in and out of the bath and nurse should ensure that every patient can summon help easily if he feels ill or faint. If the bathroom is not fitted with a bell, a handbell can be placed on a stool beside the bath and nurse should not leave the patient indefinitely without making sure that all is well.

Bathing in Bed

Those patients who are unable to go to the bath are washed all over whilst lying in bed. Again, some patients may be able to do most of this for themselves, whilst others will want the whole attention of one or two nurses. To give a patient a bath in this way, the windows are closed and the curtains are drawn.

The toilet requisites are in the patient's locker and a plentiful supply of hot water is brought to the bedside. The top bed-clothes are removed and the patient is arranged between two blankets or towels. The one under the patient is to protect the bed from drips and splashes whilst the top one covers the patient apart from the part actually being washed. It is wise to have a plan when washing a patient otherwise it is easy to wash some parts twice and other parts not at all. Most nurses start with the face, using one flannel either with or without soap as the patient prefers. The rest of the body is washed with another flannel, which is well soaped so that a good lather is obtained. The soap is rinsed off carefully and thorough drying is essential. Folds and clefts of the body must be scrupulously washed and the patient will appreciate being able to put his hands and feet into the water if nurse holds the bowl so that he may do so.

This bath gives the nurse an excellent opportunity of observing the general state and physical condition of the patient. She should also seize this opportunity to let the patient talk to her. If two nurses are attending to the patient they must resist the temptation to talk to one another whilst washing and drying the person between them. Nothing could be more unfriendly or demoralising to the patient than to feel he is simply an object which has to be cleaned. When the bath is finished the patient is given clean clothes which have been warming on a nearby radiator, the bed is made, and the patient made comfortable. Toilet articles are replaced in their proper place in the locker and the bath sheets or blankets are also put away.

Bathing can be done either in the morning or the evening. At other times the hands and face should be washed, and all patients should be allowed to wash their hands after using the bedpan or commode.

Care of Nails and Hair

Nails should be attended to at regular intervals. Many women can file their own finger nails, but if not, the nurse should do it. Toe nails must be kept short and cut straight across. In some diseases, notably diabetes mellitus, the feet need professional attention and a chiropodist may attend the patient in the ward.

Hair should be kept well brushed and combed, long hair should be arranged in the style the patient prefers. Long-stay patients need to have their hair washed and this is sometimes undertaken by nurses though many hospitals have visiting hairdressers.

A man who is too ill to attend to his own personal toilet will be bothered and distressed by the growth of his beard. Many wards for male patients have a visiting barber who performs this service. Convalescent patients are often extremely helpful to their more ill colleagues, but if neither of these is available the nurse can shave the patient quite easily. Most wards have an electric razor which makes the procedure of shaving a straight-forward one. If no electric razor is available, nurse should use a safety razor with a new blade together with an adequate supply of shaving soap and really hot water.

Care of the Teeth and Mouth

Most people clean their teeth when they have a bath or a wash and the same service should be carried out for the patient. Those patients well enough to go to the bathroom will look after their own teeth. Those who are being bathed in bed but who can still look after their own personal hygiene need to be provided with a beaker of water and a receiver in which to spit. They will have their own brush and tooth paste in the locker. The really helpless patients need to have their mouths cleaned for them. The requirements for this are put on a tray which is brought to the bedside.

Requirements for a Tray for Cleaning the Mouth

    Moist swabs
    Forceps with clip to carry the swabs
    Solutions: Sodium Bicarbonate, 1 teaspoonful to a pint of
             water
             Mouth Wash
             Liquid Paraffin
    Receiver for used instruments
    Paper bag for dirty swabs
    Paper towel to protect bedclothes

The actual cleaning is done with swabs held in forceps. The swabs are moistened by being dipped in a solution of sodium bicarbonate; mucus dissolves in this solution and cleaning is therefore easier. Plenty of swabs should be used, all thoroughly moist. The teeth and all the surfaces of the gums and cheeks must receive this attention, as well as the tongue. When the mouth is clean it should be swabbed over with a pleasant-tasting mouth wash and some grease applied to the lips to prevent cracking. The patient who is ill and helpless enough to receive this attention will require it frequently. The more often it is done, the easier it is to do, and the mouth is kept in a much more pleasant condition. Two-hourly attention is needed in some cases.

Dentures

Many patients wear dentures and the very ill must have their teeth cleaned for them. The patient removes them and puts them in a bowl. Nurse takes them to the bathroom and brushes them under running cold water, using a denture brush. It is sometimes necessary to use toothpaste as well. Nurses must handle dentures carefully. They may break if they are dropped into a wash basin and the shape of some can be altered if they are put into hot water. If patients prefer to sleep without their dentures they should be cleaned and then placed in a denture bath of water or solution such as *Steradent* which is kept in the locker; they must be rinsed in clean water before use. Dentures should never be left in the mouth of an unconscious patient. There is a very real danger that they may slip down into the larynx and cause asphyxia.

Nurses should never begrudge time spent on the personal hygiene of the patient. However ill a patient is, he feels refreshed and generally better after a nurse has attended to his bodily cleanliness and comfort. Patients do not always appreciate a doctor's skill, but they never forget the dexterity and kindness of the nurse who keeps them clean.

FURTHER READING

Cairney, J. *The Human Body.* Peryer (N.Z.)
Ross and Wilson, *Foundations of Anatomy and Physiology.* Livingstone.
Rowett, *Basic Anatomy and Physiology.* Murray.

CHAPTER 6

THE NURSE AND THE PATIENT'S COMFORT—THE BODY FRAMEWORK

When considering the bodily comfort of the patient it is helpful to consider the underlying structures of the body and their functions. The body has a jointed framework of bone which provides support and gives attachment for the muscles which move it. Other parts of the skeleton or framework are adapted to give protection to vital organs and attachment to the large sheets of muscles which bound the abdominal cavity.

The central supporting pole of the structure is the vertebral column, which, because it is jointed for almost the entire length, provides extreme flexibility and yet can be held rigid by the muscles which cross each of its many joints. It also protects the vital cables of nerves along which messages pass to and from the brain. Above the vertebral column is the skull, a bony box in which the brain lies safely enclosed, its citadel only breached by the points of entry of incoming sensation, the ear, the eye, and the vital cable of the spinal cord itself. The shoulder girdle is joined to the central framework, and below this the ribs provide a protective cage for the heart and by their movement cause air to be sucked in and out of the lungs. The pelvic girdle shields and protects the uterus from injury and provides a stable joint where the lower limbs join the trunk.

The joints of this framework which are strongly bound with ligaments are enclosed in capsules whose inner linings secrete lubricating fluid. Movement of all joints is brought about by muscles which pass across them, usually arranged in groups of two or more. Thus one may cause the joint to bend while another causes it to straighten. Over the muscles and under the skin is a layer of connective tissue and fat, thicker in some places than others, and where the body is subject to undue pressure and friction the skin itself may be specially thick and tough.

Prevention of Pressure Sores

When a patient is nursed in bed certain problems arise. He puts abnormal pressure on parts of his body not designed to with-

stand it. If this pressure is sufficient to cut off the blood supply
to the underlying tissues they will die and the skin over the area
will ulcerate. Diagrams show the areas subject to special pressure
when the patient is lying on his back, his side or sitting up. All
sorts of preventive measures may be employed to reduce pressure, starting with the choice of a suitable mattress. Sorbo-

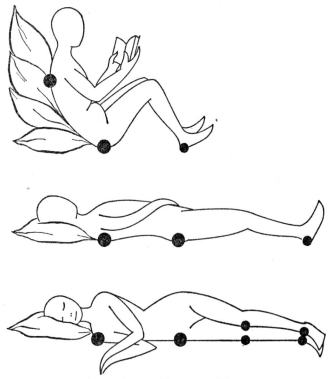

FIG. 2   Areas subject to special pressure

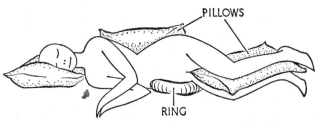

FIG. 3   Pillows placed to relieve pressure

rubber mattresses are soft and comfortable, but if the patient is very heavy an alternating pressure bed may be used. This is made of corrugated polythene and alternate sections are inflated and deflated by an electric pump, thus reducing the pressure on one area for short periods of time. If these mattresses are not available sorbo or air-cushions are useful and old-fashioned water pillows, though cumbersome, are comfortable. Some patients are nursed on sheepskins (real or synthetic). These prevent the patient from slipping down the bed and are warm and cosy to lie on.

For preventing pressure on heels, knees and ankles, frequent turning of the patient is essential. Sheepskin heel pads are very effective. The methods of placing pillows to relieve pressure are illustrated. It should be remembered that any pads or pillows used must be removed and replaced regularly. With patients who are a special risk, those who are paralysed for example, specially designed mattresses are used (see page 196). Keeping the skin in good condition and the sheets taut and smooth all help to prevent soreness and discomfort. Nurses must be very watchful when dealing with incontinent patients, cleansing and drying their buttocks as soon as they become wet. Careful drying and frequent turning have been proved to be the most effective method of preventing soreness.

Posture

As the patient lies in bed his muscles become weak from disuse. If one muscle becomes weak and another retains its power the joint may be pulled unevenly and lie in an unnatural position. This may weaken it or cause it to stiffen in an abnormal way, making it difficult to use it afterwards without a long series of special exercises. It is very important that the joints the patient is not moving should be supported at all times in the so-called neutral position (one between the two extremes of movement of which the joint is capable), and that all the natural curves of the spine should be preserved. In some cases it is more important to preserve the natural body alignment than in others. In patients with fractures, for example, the whole mattress, or part of it, is supported by boards placed over the bed springs to stop the patient from slipping into a bad position.

Prevention of 'foot drop'

One of the most important deformities caused by simply resting in bed is 'foot drop' (see Fig. 4) and for this reason all patients who are in bed for any length of time should have support to their feet as illustrated, and the weight of the bedclothes taken by a cradle. A soft light blanket placed next to the patient will keep him warm under the cradle. Overstretching of joints such as the knee joint may be prevented by the use of small sorbo-pads, and excessive flexion of joints by regular straightening. For

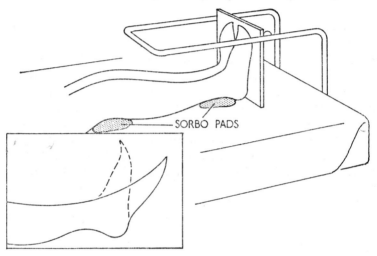

SORBO PADS

FIG. 4 Prevention of 'foot drop'

example, undue flexion of the hip in a patient nursed for many weeks in a sitting position may be prevented by lying the patient flat for a short time every day. Any joint the patient cannot move himself should be gently exercised for him by the nurse or physiotherapist every day. Painful limbs can always be supported on pillows, though in some cases it may be necessary to make special splints for their support

Respiration

Another point to be considered is that the patient must at all times be able to expand his chest wall and draw air easily into his lungs. If the lungs are not fully expanded fluid tends to collect in the lung tissue and there is a risk of infection. If the patient sits up with his shoulders falling forward, the natural movement of his rib cage is impeded and his lungs do not fully expand.

One of the best positions for free chest expansion is flat on the back, but if the patient cannot breathe lying down or fluid is being drained from the pleural space, he must sit up. Nurses should encourage deep breathing every time they make the patient's bed and make sure his back is firmly supported.

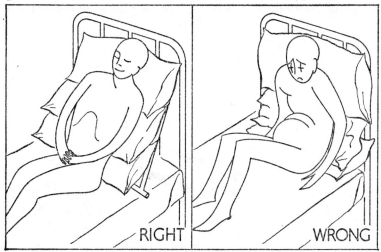

RIGHT   WRONG

FIG. 5 Sitting up in bed

Circulation

When the patient lies still his circulation tends to become sluggish and there is a risk of blood clots forming in the veins of the legs. This is dangerous as these clots may move to the lungs (pulmonary embolus) and cause a fatal collapse. Undue pressure from supporting pillows and slings may also interfere with the circulation. Regular movement and exercising of the patient's limbs prevent clot formation.

Bearing these points in mind the patient may be nursed in any position that the doctor orders, or that is comfortable to him. A few of the most commonly used positions are mentioned below:

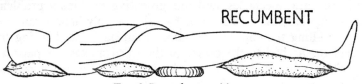

RECUMBENT

FIG. 6 Recumbent position

Recumbent (flat on the back) (see Fig. 6)

This position is not often used and is not very comfortable for the patient, as it is very difficult for him to eat, drink or use a bedpan or urinal. He finds it tiring to hold a book or write, and has a very limited view of the ward and his neighbours. The diagram shows the best way to place the pillows in the bed. An

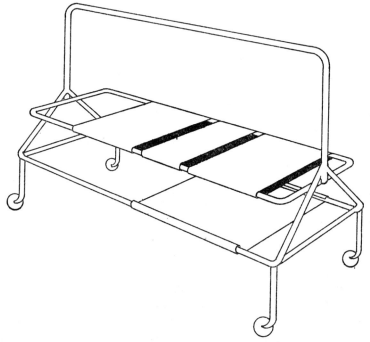

FIG. 7 Stryker frame (turning mechanism and upper section not shown)

alternative is to nurse the patient on a frame such as the *Stryker* frame which makes it possible, by removing a special sling, to slide a bedpan under the patient without moving him. The difficulty of reading in this position can be overcome by the use of prismatic spectacles, and though eating remains a problem, drinking is made much easier by using a polythene straw and never filling the cup or glass more than half full. Turning the head of the bed to the centre of the ward makes the patient's position more social, but may lead to difficulties with reading lamps and plugs.

Prone and Semi-prone (*flat on the face*)

The patient is placed as shown. This position is often used for unconscious patients as they are less likely to choke and inhale their secretions when face downwards. If the patient is con-

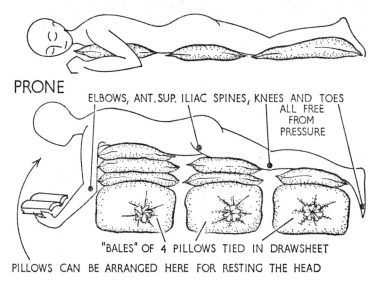

PRONE

ELBOWS, ANT. SUP. ILIAC SPINES, KNEES AND TOES ALL FREE FROM PRESSURE

"BALES" OF 4 PILLOWS TIED IN DRAWSHEET

PILLOWS CAN BE ARRANGED HERE FOR RESTING THE HEAD

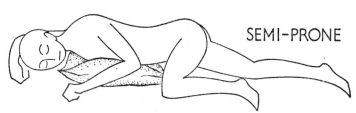

SEMI-PRONE

Fig. 8 Prone and semi-prone positions

scious and the position is being used to give him a change of view or relieve the pressure on his back, he can be raised on pillows as shown, which leaves his hands free. The *Stryker* frame can easily be turned in to a face-down position also.

Semi-recumbent

This is a very comfortable position and frequently used. The patient can see around him, and there is no undue pressure on his sacral area or heels.

Sitting Up

This position is often necessary either to aid drainage from the chest or abdominal cavity or to make it easier for the patient to breathe. He may be kept sitting up as shown, or in a special adjustable bed which winds into an armchair position and is often used for patients with heart disease who find difficulty

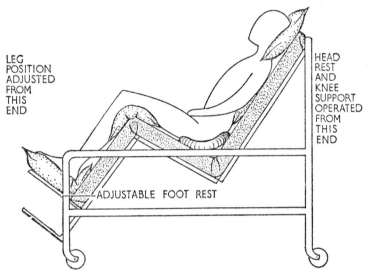

LEG
POSITION
ADJUSTED
FROM
THIS
END

HEAD
REST
AND
KNEE
SUPPORT
OPERATED
FROM
THIS
END

ADJUSTABLE FOOT REST

FIG. 9 The adjustable bed

in breathing. If preferred, the patient may actually be nursed in a chair and may find it more comfortable than a bed. If he is nursed in a bed the pillows require expert placing if he is not to sit hunched forward, and his locker and bedtable should be pulled well forward so that he may reach them with the minimum of effort. Some people prefer to sleep sitting up and resting forwards on a pillow on their bedtable.

Head up or Head down

If desired the foot or head of the bed may be raised on blocks. The 'head up' position may be used when a patient who must lie flat is having difficulty in breathing, it also helps to promote drainage from the kidneys. The 'head down' position is used when the blood pressure is low to bring blood to the brain and heart, or drain secretions from the mouth if the patient cannot swallow normally.

Change of Position

Whatever position is decided upon, the more helpless the patient, the more frequently he must be turned; in many cases it may be necessary to change his position every hour. Most patients have their beds made twice a day, when clean linen is given as needed. The draw sheet is removed and replaced and all pillows are taken out, plumped up and rearranged. During the making of the bed the patient should feel that he is the centre of interest and attention, not a mindless log rolled between two

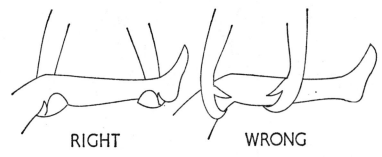

RIGHT   WRONG

FIG. 10 Supporting a limb

nurses. He should be encouraged to help himself as much as possible, using an overbed handle to lift himself if he can. Undue exposure should be avoided or he will be tired and chilled after the bed is made. If the patient is helpless the nurse must handle his limbs with the greatest care, supporting the joints gently from below and making sure that his head does not fall back. When rolling the patient from side to side a firm grasp of his shoulder and hip make it easier to move him. When he has been settled in his new position all his belongings should be moved within his reach again and it is often a useful opportunity to give him a drink or refill his hot-water bottle.

If a patient has to be lifted, the easiest method is the 'Australian' lift (as illustrated). However, whichever method is used the nurse must remember to keep the weight she is lifting as near to her own centre of gravity as possible, and to bend her knees but not her back as she lifts. The secret of successful lifting is for the nurse to keep her head over her heels.

If the nurse remembers at all times that her patients run the risks of stiff joints, sore skin, chest infection and urinary infection just by lying in bed, she will make sure that they are properly

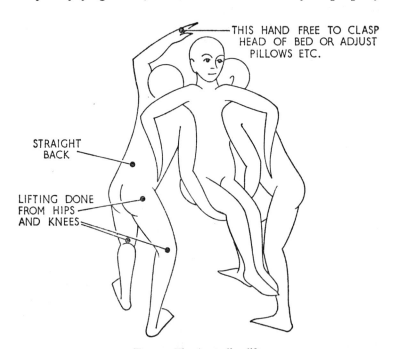

THIS HAND FREE TO CLASP HEAD OF BED OR ADJUST PILLOWS ETC.

STRAIGHT BACK

LIFTING DONE FROM HIPS AND KNEES

FIG. 11 The Australian lift

positioned, regularly turned, carefully cleansed and gently handled. She will see that they have regular breathing and leg exercises and make every effort to get them out of bed as soon as possible.

FURTHER READING

Physiotherapy Helps Nursing. Nursing Times Reprint.

Lifting Patients in Hospital. Leaflet issued by Chartered Society of Physiotherapy.

CHAPTER 7

FOOD AND THE PATIENT

All over the world people eat the food that nature has provided for them. In ancient times people ate the food that was readily available such as roots, shellfish and berries. Then someone learnt how to make a fishing net and someone else a throwing stick so that hunting and fishing added to their sources of food. Some tribes started to build up herds of animals and follow them as they wandered in search of grazing, others learnt how to till the soil and cultivate grain. Even so, if the harvest failed or was late, the whole tribe might go hungry or die of starvation. It was no coincidence that so much primitive religion and magic was concerned with the spring sowing and the harvest. Gradually as the world has grown smaller civilized people need no longer depend on the fruits of any one harvest, the spoils of the earth are literally brought to their tables. At one meal there may be oranges from Spain, sugar from the West Indies, bacon from Denmark and tea from Sri Lanka. At the same time, on the other side of the world, someone in a less prosperous community may be dying of hunger. Yet it is only very recently that much attention has been paid to the problems of equal distribution of food. In England during the second world war, when rationing was a necessity, a deliberate attempt was made to provide proper nutrition for those groups of the population, such as children and expectant mothers, whose need was the greatest. This has continued to a limited degree in the provision of special food such as milk and vitamins at infant welfare clinics, and the provision of milk and hot dinners at school. The World Health Organization is also involved with the problem of a more equal distribution of world food resources.

FOOD IN THE BODY

Wherever one lives and whatever one eats there are certain basic factors in food which are necessary to the body to enable its cells and tissues to function properly. Food taken into the body is broken down, absorbed and used to provide heat and energy, to repair and replace body tissues, and to provide the

D

raw material for those substances such as enzymes, which regu-
late bodily processes. The body possesses a unique assembly
line stretching from the mouth to the anus, where food is taken
in, broken down both physically and chemically, in preparation

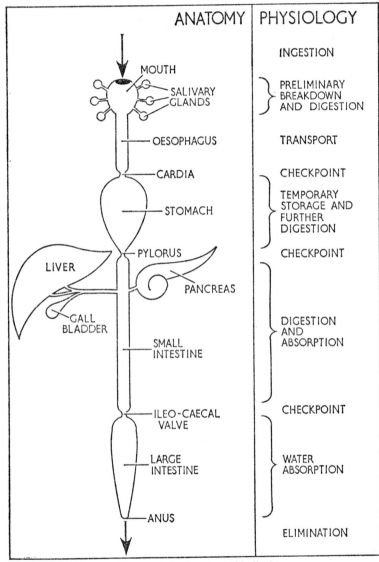

ANATOMY	PHYSIOLOGY
	INGESTION
MOUTH	
SALIVARY GLANDS	PRELIMINARY BREAKDOWN AND DIGESTION
OESOPHAGUS	TRANSPORT
CARDIA	CHECKPOINT
STOMACH	TEMPORARY STORAGE AND FURTHER DIGESTION
PYLORUS	CHECKPOINT
LIVER PANCREAS GALL BLADDER SMALL INTESTINE	DIGESTION AND ABSORPTION
ILEO-CAECAL VALVE	CHECKPOINT
LARGE INTESTINE	WATER ABSORPTION
ANUS	ELIMINATION

FIG. 12 A 'unique assembly line'

for its absorption into the blood and lymphatic systems, and the unused waste passed out of the body. Arrangements are made for the newly absorbed foodstuffs to be carried directly to the liver for further chemical action and they are then distributed all over the body in the bloodstream, ready to be used by the cells. Like any thrifty housewife the body also has several storage depots, carbohydrates are stored as glycogen in the liver, and fat is deposited in various sites. One of these storage depots is behind the eye which explains why in starvation the eyes appear sunken.

Each part of the alimentary tract has its own function for which it is particularly adapted:

The Mouth

Here food is broken up by the action of chewing, moistened by saliva and acted upon by an enzyme (see table at the end of the chapter). It is then passed into the oesophagus.

The Oesophagus

This is a hollow tube which acts as a conveyor belt taking food from the mouth to the stomach. A ring (sphincter) muscle at the lower end prevents the regurgitation of food from the stomach.

The Stomach

This is a hollow distensible bag which acts as a reservoir for food, holding it for several hours while it is churned and acted upon by acid and enzymes. The lower end of the stomach is also guarded by a sphincter.

The Small Intestine

This is a long tube, many feet in length, coiled and slung in the abdominal cavity. Many glands within its walls produce digestive juices. Associated glands, the liver and the pancreas, pour their secretions into it. The whole surface is adapted for maximum absorption, being thrown into folds and covered with multitudes of tiny projections, like a piece of ruched velvet. It is through these tiny projections, or villi, that absorption takes place, and no food can be used by the body until it has been so absorbed. Waste matter passes on into the large intestine.

At the lower end of the small intestine is the ileo-caecal valve which prevents this material from regurgitating.

The Large Intestine

This extends from the ileo-caecal valve to the rectum and it is here that water is absorbed and the remaining waste passed on to be excreted.

Control of the Alimentary Tract

Food is passed the whole length of the alimentary tract by the action of two sets of muscles which are controlled by the autonomic nervous system. Glandular secretions are also beyond any conscious control. Thus emotion may affect digestion, for the effect of fear and anger on the autonomic system is to allow the sympathetic to act at the expense of the parasympathetic. The person who says he is 'sick with fright' is speaking more truly than he knows. Similarly when children say something has 'made their mouths water' they are saying that the glandular secretions in the alimentary tract may be stimulated by the taste, the smell or even the appearance of delicious food. Appetising food is therefore digested more efficiently because although it is not always realised, the stomach 'waters' when the mouth does.

Types of Nutrients

There are five different types of nutrients:
    Proteins
    Carbohydrates
    Fats
    Minerals
    Vitamins
Water is also required.

Energy Value of Food

Each person needs food to provide him with heat and energy so that he may carry out the normal processes of living. The energy value of foods is reckoned in units called Calories, and just as a coin in the gas meter will give four hours worth of heat and light, so scientists have calculated how much energy will be gained from known quantities of certain foods. Food is burnt in the body in the same way as gas is consumed in the gas fire with the important difference that light is not emitted! Using the scientists' tables it is possible to calculate the energy value of every mouthful of food that is eaten. Calories can be obtained from all foods and individual Calorific requirements differ. There are several reasons for this, the most important being that no two people burn their body fuel at the same rate. Some burn slowly like a stove with the 'damper in', others burn rapidly with the 'damper out'; the regulating factor in this case being the thyroid gland. The more physical work a person does the more Calories he burns, thus nurses need a higher Calorie intake than those whose job is more sedentary, and they both need more than the patient who is lying in bed all day. Age, sex and possibly climate are other factors which affect Calorie requirements. If Calories are constantly taken in excess of energy requirements the extra food taken is converted into fat and stored in the fat depots, as many people know to their cost.

Types of Nutrients

Proteins. These may be of animal or vegetable origin, and their prime function is for growth and repair, though they provide some energy and on occasion can be broken down and used as fat. Foods rich in protein are meat, fish, cheese and eggs. They must all be broken down into amino acids before they can be absorbed. They are then built again into the types of protein the body needs. One gram of protein gives approximately four Calories.

Carbohydrates. These consist of sugars and starches. They provide heat and energy, but any surplus may be deposited as fat. Foods rich in carbohydrates are sugar, bread, potatoes and cereals. They must all be broken down into glucose before they can be absorbed. One gram of carbohydrate gives approximately four Calories.

Fats. These may be of animal or vegetable origin and their function is to provide heat and energy. Foods rich in fat are margarine, butter, fat meat and dairy produce. They must be broken down into fatty acids and glycerol before absorption. One gram of fat gives approximately nine Calories.

Minerals. These include Sodium, Potassium, Magnesium, Sulphur, Iodine, Copper, Calcium, Phosphorus and Iron dissolved in the various body fluids. They are vital for many different reasons. Calcium and Phosphorus are necessary for strong bones and teeth; Iron for normal blood cells; Sodium and Potassium are necessary in their correct proportions to control the fluid balance of the body.

Vitamins. These accessory food factors are also vital to life and their functions and sources are set out in a table at the end of the chapter.

Water. Water is essential for all bodily processes, acting as a solvent for all chemicals and enzymes. It forms two-thirds of the body tissue.

Planning a Diet

To build an adequate diet from the various nutrients three things are important.

Building foods should be represented each day. By 'building foods' is meant those that build and maintain the skeleton, for example, calcium; those that build the muscles, *e.g.*, protein; and those that build the components of the blood, *e.g.*, iron.

Protective foods, those that contain vitamins and

Energy foods, those which are good sources of fat and carbohydrates, must also be included.

Appetite should determine the amount of energy foods that are taken, although it should be noted that appetite can be affected by emotional factors.

Nutrition in illness

When a patient is ill the problem of his nutrition becomes of vital importance. He is weak and tired and has lost his appetite just at the time when it is important to him to keep up his intake of protective and building foods to help him in his recovery. Worse still, he may be unconscious, or have actual difficulty in chewing and swallowing. Just at this time when tasty home-made dishes might tempt him, he is in hospital where the food must of necessity be bought and served as in any catering establishment, and it is not easy to consider individual preferences. Here the nurse comes into her own. If she obeys a few simple rules she will make a great deal of difference to the way her patient enjoys his meals.

No other activity should be taking place in the ward during the serving of meals, and the nurse should see that all sanitary needs have been attended to, and utensils cleared away, before the meal is served. First of all the patient must be placed in a comfortable position and arranged so that he may feed himself if possible. Next, the tray which is brought to the bed-side should be spotlessly clean, and the food should be really hot if it is intended to be. This is a problem which has never been really successfully solved in hospital; no one has yet devised a method of keeping a hot trolley really hot, and most of the food has to be reheated in the ward. An alternative is to have the patient's tray sent up from a central kitchen, but this also creates difficulties as it does away with the personal service to the patient by the nurse who knows him and his condition at the moment the meal is being served. It is im-portant that the second course is never placed on the tray until the patient has finished his first course. It is better to give small portions and give out second helpings as required. Lastly, it is important that the nurse should remember any little personal fads and fancies of the patient – does he take sugar? does he like skin? does he take custard? is the state of his teeth such that he would prefer soft food?

Feeding the Patient

Some patients are unable to feed themselves and the nurse must be prepared to feed them. This is a simple job but one which, if skilfully performed, makes a great deal of difference to the patient's well-being. The secret of success is not to appear hurried but to draw up a chair close to the bed and feed the patient in a leisurely manner. It is as well to remember that patients being fed are unlikely to be able to talk, so that conversation, if any, should be a monologue for the nurse. When the meal is over the patient might appreciate a mouth-wash immediately, rather than waiting until later.

The patient who is unconscious must, of course, be fed by another route, because he has no swallowing reflex, and any food placed in his mouth might pass into his respiratory passages and choke him.

Feeding through a Tube

One method is by a tube passed through the nose or mouth into the stomach. The size of the tube depends upon which of these routes is chosen. It may be made of either rubber or polythene, the latter having the advantage of being less irritant and can therefore be left in position for longer periods. If the patient is conscious the procedure is explained to gain his co-operation. He is assured that it is not painful and that the discomfort he may feel in swallowing the tube is only temporary. If able, he will blow his nose and remove his dentures. If the patient can sit up in bed the passage of the tube is easier.

REQUIREMENTS

Tray containing:

Bowl of water in which there is a nasal tube and feeding funnel.

60 ml of water in a medicine glass. Syringe and litmus paper for testing. The prepared and warmed feed in a jug.

(The temperature of the feed may be taken in the kitchen).

Spigot and strapping (if the tube is to remain in position).

Technique

The bedding and the patient's clothing are protected. The tube is wetted and passed into a nostril. If one side presents difficulties the other may be easier (sometimes the septum is not in the midline). The patient is asked to swallow and to keep on doing so as the tube is passed. If the nurse has a mental picture of the length of the tube and she compares it with the size of the patient, she will have an idea of when it is in the stomach.

There are various tests for checking that the tube is in the stomach and not in the lungs.

(a) On aspirating the tube with a syringe a little gastric juice is removed if it is in the stomach; this fluid may be tested with the litmus paper. A red reaction shows the acid reaction of the stomach.

(b) If the end of the tube is placed under water, bubbles of air would indicate that it was in the lungs.

As an added precaution, thirty ml of water are passed through the tube before the feed. If the patient coughs, or becomes blue in the face, the tube must be withdrawn.

The feed at a temperature of 38°C (100°F) may be run in through the funnel, taking about ten minutes for 200 ml. The funnel is not allowed to empty, as pockets of air will cause the patient pain. After the feed a small quantity of water is poured through the tube to clear it. It may then be withdrawn, or left in position, as required. The feed is recorded in the usual way on the fluid chart.

As only a small volume of feed may be given at any one time, the feeds should be frequent, and their Calorie value carefully calculated. The doctor will usually order the amount, and the feeds are made up for twenty-four hours containing the correct Calorie value as well as the proper proportions of all the other nutrients. Proteins, carbohydrates, fats, minerals and vitamins must all be included either as fresh material or by using one of the prepared feeds such as *Complan*. By feeding patients in this way it is possible to keep them alive and well for long periods of time.

ENZYMES OF THE DIGESTIVE TRACT

	Name	*Action*
Mouth	Ptyalin	Cooked starch to dextrin and maltose
Stomach	Pepsin with Hydrochloric Acid	Proteins to peptones.
	Rennin	Curdles caseinogen.
Pancreas	Amylase	Starch to dextrin and maltose.
	Lipase	Fats to fatty acids and glycerol (in presence of bile).
	Tripsinogen	When acted on by enterokinase to become tripsin, turns proteins to amino acids.
Intestine	Enterokinase	(See above.)
	Erepsin.	Proteins to amino acids.
	Maltase Invertase Lactase	Reduces sugars to their simplest forms e.g., glucose, laevulose and galactose.
Liver	Bile	Helps the action of lipase

FUNCTIONS AND SOURCES OF VITAMINS

Vitamin	*Function*	*Common Sources*
A	To preserve healthy skin and mucous membrane. It also helps to keep the cornea normal and is needed to make visual purple.	Halibut and cod liver oils. Butter (and margarine). Coloured vegetables (lettuce, tomato, etc.) contain carotene which the body can turn into Vitamin A.

Shortage of Vitamin A reduces resistance to respiratory infection. Severe shortage causes a serious condition of the cornea, xerophthalmia.

FUNCTIONS AND SOURCES OF VITAMINS—*Continued*

Vitamin	*Function*	*Common Sources*
B1. Aneurin Thiamin	To help in carbohydrate metabolism To keep nerve tissues healthy	Cereals Yeast. Marmite. Offal (liver, kidney, etc.)

Shortage of Vitamin B1 may cause neuritis.
Severe shortage causes a condition called beri-beri.

B2. Riboflavine Nicotinic acid	To help in the normal function of the skin and intestinal tract.	Cereals. Yeast. Offal.

Shortage of riboflavine causes a sore mouth and tongue.
Shortage of nicotinic acid causes a condition called pellagra.

B6 Pyridoxine	To help in protein metabolism	Cereals. Yeast Eggs

B12 Cyanocobalamin	To help make red blood cells	Liver.

Inability to absorb Vitamin B12 causes pernicious anaemia.

C
Ascorbic acid
	To aid growth of bone and the
	healing of wounds.
		Fresh fruits,
		  especially citrus
		  fruits.
		Potatoes.

Shortage of Vitamin C causes scurvy.

D	To help in the growth of healthy bones and teeth	Fish liver oils. Dairy products. Margarine.

Shortage of Vitamin D causes rickets.

FURTHER READING

Brown, Ann M., *Practical Nutrition for Nurses.* Heinemann Medical Books.
Childe, Gordon, *What Happened in History.* Pelican.
Drummond and Wilbraham, *Manual of Nutrition.* H.M.S.O.

CHAPTER 8

THE PATIENT'S WATER
REQUIREMENTS AND FLUID BALANCE

A healthy young man weighing 70 kilograms (11 stones) has about 43 litres (75 pints) of water in his body. BODY FLUID is the name given to this water and its dissolved substances. It is found in two situations:

 1. INTRACELLULAR FLUID—in the actual cells of the body, being held within the wall or membrane of each cell, and

 2. EXTRACELLULAR FLUID—outside the cells of the body.

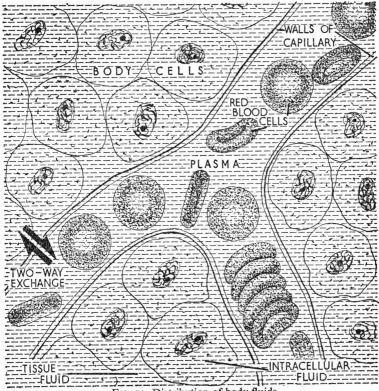

FIG. 13 Distribution of body fluids

Extracellular Fluid is:

(a) the fluid part of the blood (the plasma),
(b) the fluid which lies in the spaces between the cells—interstitial fluid, or tissue fluid—(both names are used),
(c) the fluids that are separated from the plasma in a special kind of way, *i.e.*

Serous fluids from the serous membranes
Digestive juices in the alimentary tract
Cerebro-spinal fluid in and around the brain, and spinal cord
Aqueous and vitreous humours of the eye
Synovial fluid in the joints
Urine in the kidneys.

Water and some dissolved substances pass through the cell

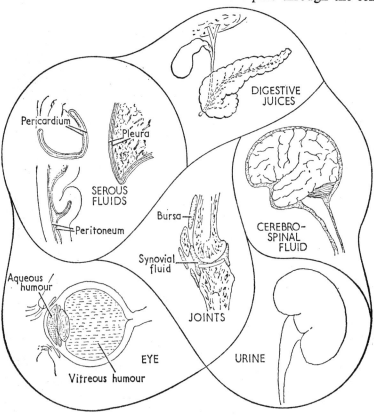

FIG. 14 Extracellular fluids

membranes, whilst other dissolved substances are kept out. This balance is controlled by the concentration of salts in the water, especially the salts of Sodium (Na) and Potassium (K). These salts carry an electrical charge, and for this reason are often referred to as ELECTROLYTES.

Water can be taken into the body in many ways.

Normally water is taken in by the mouth, and is absorbed into the body from the stomach, small and large intestines.

Artificially it can be given subcutaneously, intravenously or rectally.

Water is passed out of the body from the kidneys as urine,

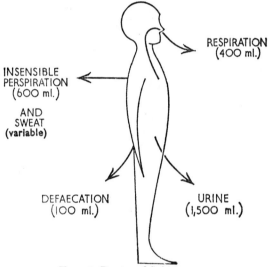

FIG. 15 Routes of fluid loss

from the skin as insensible perspiration and sweat, and in the expired air from the lungs. A little is passed in the faeces from the large intestine.

Every day about 1,500 *millilitres are taken in* as water, and 1,000 millilitres in food, depending upon the kind of food. Watery foods like lettuce and fresh ripe fruit will obviously contain more water than bread and cake. As the cells of the body burn up the foodstuffs in the presence of oxygen, they form about 300 millilitres of water.

Every day about 1,500 *millilitres are passed out* as urine, but this varies with the fluid taken in. About 600 millilitres are excreted as insensible perspiration constantly, but the amount of sweat varies according to the temperature of the environment, the muscular activity of the body, and even the amount and kind of clothing worn. About 400 millilitres are given out in respiration, and 100 millilitres in defaecation.

Although water intake may drop to nothing, leaving only the amount from the burning up of foodstuffs in the cells, the

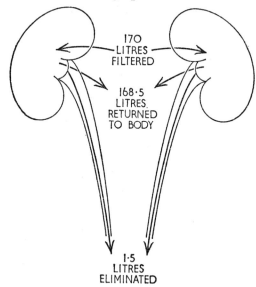

170
LITRES
FILTERED

168·5
LITRES.
RETURNED
TO BODY

1·5
LITRES
ELIMINATED

FIG. 16 Passage of fluid through the kidneys

output cannot be reduced to nothing. What is more difficult to appreciate is that although the water intake may cease, there is always some fluid to be excreted. Insensible perspiration and the water vapour from the lungs never fall below 1,000 millilitres a day, and from 400 to 500 millilitres of urine are essential for elimination of waste products. If fluid is not taken in to cover this loss, the condition of DEHYDRATION occurs.

The Turnover of Fluid Inside the Body is vast. There is a constant to and fro interchange between the plasma and the interstitial fluid. One startling example is that almost 170 litres of fluid are filtered through the kidneys in 24 hours. About 168·5 litres are reabsorbed. The approximate difference of 1·5 litres is passed as urine.

Cells Everywhere are bathed in interstitial fluid (tissue fluid) in order that nourishing substances and oxygen can pass into them. This tissue fluid seeps through the capillary walls from the closed circuit of the bloodstream. When it has been used by the cells, excess fluid and waste substances are taken up by a different kind of capillary (lymphatic capillary) which interweaves between the cells. This changed fluid is now called lymph, and is moved from lymphatic capillaries to lymphatic vessels. Before it is finally emptied into ducts, it passes through lymphatic glands. Lymphatic glands make lymphocytes, a kind of white blood cell, and these are added to the lymph.

In the event of cell inflammation they also remove bacteria from the lymph. The filtered lymph is emptied from two ducts, the thoracic duct, and the right lymphatic duct, into the blood stream.

Disturbances of Fluid Balance. Patients may be admitted to hospital with signs of insufficient intake of fluid. These signs may be thirst, or a dry tongue, and there may be a history of passing only very little urine (oliguria). The patients may have:

(*a*) been too weak to bother to take fluids, or unable because of being unconscious;

(*b*) pain, or an obstruction in the mouth, throat, or oesophagus;

(*c*) been stranded on a desert island, or just neglected by those around them.

Other patients may be admitted to hospital with signs of having put out too much fluid. They may be passing large quantities of urine (polyuria), or there may be a history of vomiting or diarrhoea.

Fluid Charts. It is necessary in some instances to have a record showing how much fluid the patient takes in and how much fluid he puts out. This record is made on an intake and output chart, and notes must be made of the amounts of fluid which enter and leave the body, and the routes they take. The type of fluid should be noted—tap water, normal saline, vomit, urine, for example.

Charts must be filled in accurately and Arabic numerals should be used (1, 2, 3, 4, etc.). In most hospitals the amounts are measured in millilitres (another name is cubic centimetres), and for writing them down, ink is preferred. It is usual to total the amount of fluid at the end of either twelve or twenty-four hours according to the doctor's wishes.

There are several ways in which entries can be made. Confusion arises sometimes on the intake side. A good way to avoid confusion is to enter the amount on the chart, in the appropriate column, when it has entered the patient. For example, a jug of water is placed on the patient's locker—it should be entered when the patient has drunk the contents. Similarly, when a bottle

FLUID CHART

DATE 1.10.74   SHEET No. 3

RECORD No: 50580 D   Male Surgical UNIT

NAME MR. ERNEST BULGER   DIAG/O.P. Repair of Hiatus Hernia

TIME	FLUID	FLUIDS IN		FLUIDS OUT			REMARKS
		ORAL	I.V. RECT.	URINE	VOMIT	ASPIR.	
0800 hrs						8 ml.	Greenish fluid aspirated
0900 hrs						20	
1000 hrs				250 ml.		8	
1100 hrs						nil	
1200 hrs						10	I.V. Dextrose saline completed. I.V. Normal saline started.
1230 hrs			1,000 ml.				
1300 hrs						8	
1400 hrs				200		12	
1500 hrs						5	
1530 hrs	Water	30 ml.				4	30 ml. water to be given orally, hourly, after each aspiration.
1600 hrs	Water	30		100		25	
1700 hrs	Water	30				20	
1800 hrs	Water	30		250		20	Clear fluid aspirated.
1845 hrs				100			
1900 hrs	Water	30				40	
2000 hrs	Water	30	1,000 ml.	300		10	I.V. Normal saline completed. I.V. Dextrose saline started.
DAY TOTAL		180 ml.	2,000 ml.	1,200 ml.		190 ml.	

C6.13

of fluid has dripped through the tubing into a vein, it should be entered on the chart. If the amount of the fluid in the jug is entered on the chart at the time of placing the jug on the locker or the bottle on the stand, inaccurate recordings might be made. The jug could be refilled, or removed, or the infusion apparatus become blocked before the contents have entered the body.

Urine, vomit, or aspirations from the stomach should be entered at the time the patient either passes urine, vomits, or the nurse withdraws the fluid.

Giving Fluids by Mouth. Normally, sufficient fluid is taken into the body by mouth to supply the body's needs. This can be done provided there is little or no vomiting, and no difficulty in swallowing. It is dangerous to give fluids by mouth to an unconscious patient. Because of the absence of the swallowing reflex the fluid may pass into the lungs. When it is not possible to give fluids orally, or when oral intake is inadequate or undesirable, other means of supplying fluids must be used. This is especially important when the fluid loss is on the increase. It is generally the doctor who determines which method should be used. The patient's condition is considered, and also the purpose for which the fluid is to be given.

Giving Fluids by Rectum. Fluid may be introduced into the body by passing a tube into the rectum. Only small amounts of solutions are absorbed rectally, and they are given slowly. Rectal infusions are used:

1. to replace fluid loss,
2. to combat shock,
3. to give nourishment when fluid cannot be taken by mouth.

If possible the bladder and rectum are emptied first.

EQUIPMENT

Bowl containing:

    Funnel, tubing, clip, connection and catheter, No. 8. French gauge.

    Jug of normal saline, 180 to 240 ml at 37°C (98°F)

    Yellow petroleum jelly

    Linen or paper squares

    Receiver for used catheter

    Paper bag for used squares

    Incontinence pad.

E

Preparation of Equipment. Clean equipment is used. To make *normal saline* one teaspoonful of salt is added to 600 ml of water. This makes 0·9% solution, and is called normal saline because it is the same concentration as that found in blood and tissue fluids.

Preparation of the Patient. The nurse explains to the patient that he is to have a small injection into his bowel, and he is asked to try to retain it. The nurse makes sure that he is not in a draught, that privacy is ensured, and that the patient is turned into the left lateral position, with the knees drawn up. The bedclothes are turned back but the patient is not exposed. The buttocks are placed on an incontinence pad along the edge of the bed. The upper leg is placed over the lower leg. If this is not possible the infusion may be given with the patient lying on his back.

Method. Fluid is passed through the funnel and tubing, to expel the air, but the catheter is nipped between the finger and thumb to prevent it emptying. The catheter is lubricated and passed through the anus for about four inches. Taking care not to allow air to enter the tubing, the funnel is filled.

About twenty minutes should be taken over this procedure, the nurse sitting on a chair by the bedside. The rate of flow is regulated by the height of the funnel above the bed. When the prescribed amount has been given, the catheter is nipped, and gently withdrawn. It is detached from the tubing and placed in the receiver. The patient is made comfortable. He will retain the fluid better if he is disturbed as little as possible. Rectal infusions may be repeated six hourly.

Continuous Rectal Infusion. A continuous method can be used when a container of normal saline is suspended from a stand. The attached tubing contains a 'drip' chamber, and the flow of fluid can be regulated by a clip. About 40 drops a minute is the usual rate. The catheter is fastened to the skin with *Sellotape*. The patient is made comfortable, bedclothes adjusted, and screens drawn back.

The amount given is noted, and eventually recorded on the fluid balance chart.

Giving Fluids Subcutaneously. Fairly large quantities of sterile normal saline can be injected into the tissues under the skin. The substance hyaluronidase (*Hyalase*) is used to assist absorption.

EQUIPMENT

Sterile pack containing:
  Two dressing towels
  Five cotton wool swabs
  One small bowl or gallipot
  Two pairs of dissecting forceps
  Two pieces of gauze dressing.
A pre-sterilised, disposable 'giving' set which consists of:
  Air inlet tube
  Bottle-piercing needle or tube
  Tubing
  'Drip' chamber
  Another piece of tubing
  Clamp
  Y connection
  Two small pieces of narrow tubing and
  Two 'intra-muscular' needles.
Bottle of lotion for cleaning the skin,
Container of sterile normal saline,
Adhesive tape, scissors,
Receiver for used instruments,
Paper bag for used swabs.

Preparation of Equipment. The trolley with the equipment is taken to the bedside. The bottle of sterile normal saline, and the packet containing the 'giving' set are opened; the dressing packet is also opened. The nurse washes and dries her hands. The 'giving' set is connected to the bottle and the tubing is filled with fluid to remove the air. The tubing is clamped, and the bottle is then suspended from a stand.

Preparation of the Patient. Having made the patient comfortable, the nurse tells the patient, if he is able to understand, that at first there will be a little discomfort, but that he will not feel a great deal of pain. The outer aspect of the thigh, or the abdomen, is exposed, and the skin is cleaned.

Method. The needles are inserted at an angle of about 30° into the subcutaneous tissues. The 'giving' set is connected and strapped in place. This apparatus needs the nurse's constant attention as the rate of flow must be carefully adjusted to the two needles. If *Hyalase* has not been added to the bottle it can be put into the tubing when it is working satisfactorily.

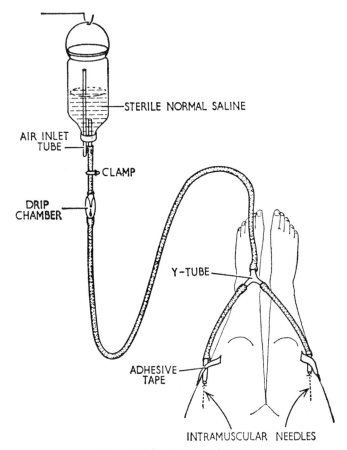

STERILE NORMAL SALINE

AIR INLET TUBE

CLAMP

DRIP CHAMBER

Y-TUBE

ADHESIVE TAPE

INTRAMUSCULAR NEEDLES

FIG. 18 Subcutaneous infusion

The patient is watched for signs of discomfort.

When the ordered amount has been given, the tubing is clamped, and the needles are withdrawn. Sterile dressings are placed over the puncture marks and secured with adhesive tape. Although this is a satisfactory method and is very useful, especially in children, it has been largely superseded by scalp vein infusion.

Equipment for Scalp Vein Infusion is similar to that for giving fluids subcutaneously, but the pre-sterilised, disposable 'giving' set is slightly different. A rigid calibrated chamber is incorporated, above the drip chamber. This helps to give exact amounts, and acts as a safety measure, if the drip should speed up unexpectedly. As only one needle is used, there is no 'Y' connection in this set.

Preparation of the Patient. A small area is shaved over the site of a selected vein. The nurse holds the head securely for the doctor.

Method. The doctor passes the needle into a superficial vein of the scalp and the tubing is connected. The needle and tubing are fastened down with adhesive tape when the fluid is dripping satisfactorily. The patient is made comfortable, and watched for signs of discomfort. When the ordered amount, generally about 30 ml. has been given, the needle is withdrawn and a sterile dressing is applied.

Giving Fluids Intravenously. Intravenous infusions of fluid are used frequently. It is possible to give large quantities of fluid in this way and it is quickly absorbed.

Solutions commonly used include blood, normal saline, glucose 5–10% in normal saline, glucose 5–10% in distilled water, plasma and synthetic 'plasma'. To most of these fluids drugs can be added if prescribed, BUT ANY CHANGE IN COLOUR; IN THE APPEARANCE OF THE FLUID, OR OF A SEDIMENT DEVELOPING, INDICATES POSSIBLE INCOMPATIBILITY. The doctor clearly states the type and amount of fluid to be given over a 24 hour period.

Equipment. The equipment is similar to that described for giving fluids subcutaneously, but the 'giving' set differs. Instead of using a Y connection, pieces of tubing and two needles, the piece of tubing from the 'drip' chamber is attached to an intravenous needle, small polythene catheter or cannula.

A sphygmomanometer will be required.

An arm splint may be required.

Preparation of Equipment. As for the subcutaneous infusion.

Preparation of the Patient. The patient is placed in a comfortable reclining position, and an explanation is given to him. The bedclothes are protected. The doctor chooses a vein which is fairly near the surface, generally on the back of the hand, or above the wrist. The sleeve of the gown, or pyjama jacket, is removed from the arm. The cuff of the sphygmomanometer is wrapped round the arm and when the doctor has washed and dried his hands, is connected to the other half of the apparatus.

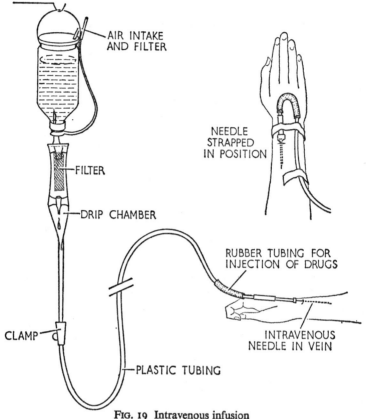

FIG. 19 Intravenous infusion

The nurse pumps the bulb of the sphygmomanometer when asked by the doctor, whilst he is cleaning the skin.

Method. The doctor passes the needle into the vein and the tubing is connected. At the same time the nurse lowers the mercury in the sphygmomanometer. The needle is fastened down with adhesive tape when the fluid is dripping satisfactorily. The patient is made comfortable.

The drips are counted with a watch. A usual speed is about 60 drips a minute.

After the required amount has been given the tubing is clamped, the needle withdrawn, and a sterile dressing applied with pressure over the site of the infusion.

If the infusion stops it may mean that the fluid is passing into

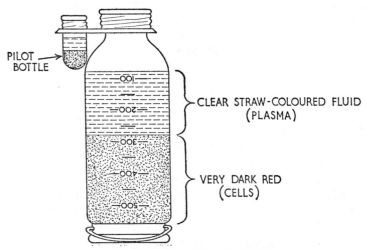

PILOT BOTTLE

CLEAR STRAW-COLOURED FLUID (PLASMA)

VERY DARK RED (CELLS)

FIG. 20 Bottle of blood (no labels shown)

the tissues. The sister in charge of the ward is informed.

Intravenous Infusion of Blood. If blood is ordered as the replacement fluid, great care is taken to make sure that it is suitable for the patient. Laboratory technicians perform grouping and cross-matching tests, and the stored blood should be allowed to stand out of the refrigerator for about two hours before it is to be used. Extreme care is necessary when checking the bottle or bag of blood and its labels, as it must be given only to the patient for whom it is prepared. Fatal consequences might result if a wrong bottle is used.

The method used is very similar to the one for giving normal saline intravenously, but a filter is incorporated in the bottle of blood.

Reactions. Although the giving of blood into a vein is regarded as a safe procedure, the nurse must still be alert for reactions. If the patient complains of:

chilliness
'chattering' teeth
pain in the loins or back,
or if there is:
increased pulse rate
dyspnoea
increased body temperature,

the sister of the ward must be told immediately. She will probably turn off the blood infusion, and inform the doctor. Throughout the procedure the pulse is recorded at half-hourly intervals, and the temperature is taken at the start, and at hourly intervals.

In some areas blood is collected into polythene bags instead of into bottles. As the bag becomes empty the sides sometimes tend to stick together, making it difficult to see the exact amount of blood in the bag and whether or not the bag needs changing. The needle may slip and pierce the side of the bag. Nurses must watch for these hazards.

The National Blood Transfusion Service. The stored blood which is used for infusions in hospitals is given freely by donors. The National Blood Transfusion Service performs the very important tasks of collecting, testing, recording and storing blood. There is a great demand for blood, and whilst donors are called upon several times, there is still a great need for healthy persons to volunteer for this contribution to the cure of disease.

Serum Hepatitis, or 'hospital' hepatitis, is a serious form of liver inflammation caused by a virus. This disease is a hazard to doctors, nurses, and technicians, and especially to nurses who are close to patients. The risk is present whenever a trace of blood from a patient carrying the virus contaminates a syringe, or a needle, or a razor, or the broken skin of any susceptible person.

Broken glassware, needle pricks, minor abrasions of hands, are all routes of transmission, and are occupational hazards of medical personnel. It can be conveyed by dialysis, by 'artificial kidney' machines.

The incubation period is long, from 50 to 160 days.

The disease is prevented by using sterile disposable equipment, and adequate sterilisation of non-disposable articles.

The patient is nursed in isolation in hospital, but there appears to be no specific treatment, or vaccination.

It is for this reason that would-be blood-donors with a history of jaundice are rejected by the National Blood Transfusion Service.

Fluids in Bottles and Bags. The labels of bottles and bags for giving fluids must be carefully checked with the doctor's prescription. It is essential for two nurses to do this

Sodium Chloride (NaCl) is prescribed by doctors and given in different preparations:

Normal saline is 0·9% solution
½ strength saline is 0·45% solution
Double strength saline is 1·8% solution

these strengths may be written:

N/S for normal, 0·9% solution
½N. for ½ strength normal, 0·45% solution
2N. for double strength normal, 1·8% solution,

as N. is used for normal.

It can be seen that mistakes could arise because of the similarity in descriptions. Nurses must be extremely careful in picking the right bottle. Substances which are not isotonic with the blood, may cause red blood cells to be severely damaged. Again, it is stressed, that two nurses must check the bottle with the doctor's prescription.

COMMON ELEMENTS

Element	Symbol	Element	Symbol
Calcium	Ca	Carbon	C
Copper	Cu	Chlorine	Cl
Iron	Fe	Nitrogen	N
Mercury	Hg	Oxygen	O
Potassium	K	Phosphorus	P
Sodium	Na	Sulphur	S
Hydrogen	H		

FURTHER READING

Bunton, *Fluid Balance Without Tears.* University College Hospital.

Kilgour, O. F. G. *An Introduction to the physical aspects of nursing science.* Heinemann.

Snively, W. D. *The Sea Within: the story of our body fluid.* Lippincott.

Taverner, *Physiology for Nurses.* E.U.P.

Warren, *Fluid Balance, Water, Salt and Blood.* Nursing Times.

CHAPTER 9

MEDICINES FOR THE PATIENT

The word 'medicine' can be used in several ways. It means 'the science and art of the treatment of disease and the maintenance of health'.

1. *Clinical medicine* is practised at the bedside of the patient where the signs and symptoms of the disease, and the progress, can be observed.
2. It can also mean 'any drug or other substances given or taken' for the purposes quoted below.
3. Nurses are often asked to 'give out the medicines'. This duty refers to the drugs prescribed by the doctor for the patient.

Uses of drugs. Drugs are substances used to cure, relieve, or prevent disease. They can be applied externally, or taken into the body. They may be extracted from plant or animal tissue, or be prepared synthetically in laboratories.

Every day new drugs are being added to the enormous number already available, and it is almost impossible for nurses and doctors to keep up to date. It is therefore of the utmost importance to all who handle drugs, to study the literature that is put forward by the various drug houses. Nursing and medical journals regularly publish lists of new drugs, and details of drugs are given in nursing care studies, and articles. It is necessary for nurses to know the expected action of the drug being used, its range of dosage, the way it has to be given to the patient, and any possible side effects.

Babies and young children, and aged patients, do not tolerate drugs at all well, so smaller doses are generally ordered for them. This also applies to patients who are underweight, but obese patients may require a dose larger than that ordered for the average adult. The actual physical condition of the patient has to be borne in mind, too.

Drugs can be used for many purposes, ranging from the replacement of insulin in diabetes mellitus, to the use of alkaline powders for neutralising extra acid secreted by the stomach in gastric ulcer. Many are used for the relief of pain, aspirin and morphine being two. rugs are alsjust Do used to combat infection, and penicillin and tetracycline are antibiotics which are frequently used.

Some drugs are used in the prevention of disease. The Sabin vaccine is given to protect against poliomyelitis, and tetanus toxoid against tetanus.

Others, barium for example, can be swallowed by a patient before the taking of a series of X-rays, and the stomach and intestines are clearly outlined.

Addiction. It is well known that certain individuals become addicted to alcohol. They feel that they cannot function properly without it, and there is a continuous craving for it. If it is withdrawn, definite symptoms may arise. Addiction occurs with drugs too. It may start quite harmlessly when sedatives are ordered, and taken by a person. Even when there is no known cause for insomnia, the person may think that he cannot sleep without them. Over a long period of time, to be effective, the dose of the drug will have to be increased.

It is for this reason that certain habit-forming drugs are controlled. The Misuse of Drugs Act ensures that the drugs are ordered, stored and given to the patient in a precise and definite way, in order that each dose of each drug thus controlled, is accurately accounted for.

Unfortunately young people become involved in drug taking in order to get 'kicks', and they often do not realise the disastrous results that eventually overtake them. It is illegal to smoke 'pot', (cannabis). It often leads to other forms of drugtaking, of which heroin is one of the most dangerous. People who become 'hooked' on heroin, i.e. find life impossible to bear without it, suffer greatly if it is withdrawn or withheld. Women heroin addicts produce babies who have heroin in their cells when they are born, and the babies are therefore addicts at birth. These mothers, as well as the babies, together with other heroin addicts will most probably die from the addiction, as there is little cure. The illegal use of Mandrax and LSD also produces disastrous results.

Propaganda, put out in different ways, encourages people to dose themselves with proprietary medicines, and often promises immediate relief of symptoms and freedom from disease. It appears to have become quite natural, therefore, to need drugs for every little ache and pain. Whenever possible self-medication is to be discouraged by nurses, otherwise this hobby will become a disease in itself. Whilst not ignoring the symptoms, those with definite signs of ill health must be persuaded to consult their own doctor.

Storage. Drugs in the solid form of pills, tablets, and capsules, are obtained from the pharmaceutical department in a variety of containers. Disposable materials such as cardboard, tinfoil and cans are used. Liquid substances, in the form of mixtures, emulsions and linctuses are found in bottles and screw-topped jars. Drugs for injections are within sealed glass ampoules and phials.

A substance is called a 'poison' if it produces injury and/or death to the person when it is introduced in sufficient amounts in, or on to, the body. There are many poisons among the drugs in the storage cupboards.

Storage Cupboards. These cupboards are placed where they are convenient to the nurses, but also out of sight of the patients, if possible.

1. *Reagent Cupboard.* The one which holds the chemical substances used in the tests carried out on urine, is generally found in the sluice annexe. It is kept locked, when not in use, as many of the chemicals are poisons.

In most wards there are three other cupboards, one for drugs and lotions for external use, one for drugs for internal use, and one for drugs controlled by the Misuse of Drugs Act.

2. *The Cupboard for Drugs and Lotions for External Use* will contain some poisons in bottles coloured dark green, dark brown or dark blue, and the bottles will be ridged. The labels will also bear the word 'poison' in red letters. 'For external use only' will be found on the label. These may be disinfectants like phenol (carbolic acid), or antiseptics like *Hibitane.*

3. *The Cupboard for Drugs for Internal Use* may have a section for drugs which are controlled by the Pharmacy and Poisons Act —those classified as Schedule 1 and 4, making them inaccessible to the public. Examples of these are the barbiturates and the sulphonamides. The law demands that a written prescription by a doctor is necessary before they can be given to a patient, that they must be clearly labelled, and kept under lock and key

in hospital. As new drugs appear very quickly and it takes time for them to be officially controlled, they may be labelled 'store as schedule 1.'

4. *The Cupboard for the Drugs Controlled by the Misuse of Drugs Act* may also include a section for Schedule drugs, if these are not contained within the cupboard for drugs for internal use. The Misuse of Drugs Act checks illicit use of some drugs of addiction. Drugs controlled in this way are:—

    a. Opium and its Derivatives.
        (*i*) papaveretum—Omnopon (containing all the alkaloids of opium)
        (*ii*) tincture of opium—Nepenthe
        (*iii*) morphine
        (*iv*) diamorphine (heroin).

    b. Cocaine in its various forms.

    c. Indian Hemp (cannabis Indica)—rarely used now.

    d. Morphine Substitutes such as:

Pethidine	Palfium
Pethilorfan	DF118 injections
Physeptone	

The cupboard may be marked 'CONTROLLED DRUGS' and is within another cupboard, being doubly locked. The keys are kept on the person of the nurse in charge of the ward or department.

In hospital the chief pharmacist is responsible for the stores of Controlled Drugs, and he keeps the main registers. A detailed record is kept of the drugs purchased and issued. They may be used in the making up of prescriptions for named patients, or by sending stock supplies to wards and departments. Each ward and department keeps a register of drugs issued to them, and how they are used. Further stocks are supplied when a satisfactory check has been made that the previous supplies have been used. A written request for the further supplies of ward stocks is sent by the sister in charge of the ward in a book provided for the purpose. They are either collected from the pharmacy by a state registered nurse, or a special messenger is allowed to deliver them to the ward. Signatures are given when the drugs are handed over.

From time to time the pharmacists visit the wards and departments and check the contents of the Controlled Drugs cupboards with the ward register, and with their registers. The
person in charge of the ward must carry out frequent checks
on these cupboards herself, too, as she is entirely responsible
for the supply entrusted to her.

(Outside hospital similar regulations are observed by chemists
and doctors and dentists, so that there is control of all the habit-
forming drugs in the country).

Drugs in hospital are kept in locked cupboards to guard against
any unknown addict from getting them and to prevent those with
suicidal tendencies from collecting them. It is also a safeguard
from dishonest visitors, and it discourages self-medication on
the part of unprofessional employees.

Prescription. Medicines for patients are prescribed by the
doctors. The patient's name must be on the form or chart used.
The doctor will write the date, the name of the drug, the amount
of each dose, and how frequently it is to be given. The method
of giving is sometimes added—by hypodermic injection, for
instance. He will add his signature or his initials. For
example:

> John Smith.
>
> 1.10.74 Morphine 15 mg. 6 hourly.
>
> (signed) R. Jones.

It is the responsibility of the nurse to carry out this written
order accurately, but if she is in any doubt at all, she must consult another nurse, or the doctor himself.

Safeguarding the Patient. To store drugs safely is not enough.
Great care must be taken when they are being given to the
patients. Whenever possible two nurses should undertake this
duty. They must concentrate on the measuring and the checking
of the drugs with the prescriptions, therefore conversation is
better avoided.

The majority of hospitals have the following practices:

General principles:

1. The equipment, and the hands of the nurse, must be
   clean.
2. Once the cupboard is unlocked the contents should
   not be left unguarded.
3. Drugs differing from the normal in colour, odour,

or consistency, should not be used.

4. In every instance the patient is identified, and the actual taking of the drug is supervised.
5. Any mistake should be reported at once to the sister in charge.

Rules concerning labels:

1. The contents of containers not clearly labelled should not be used.
2. Drugs in unmarked vessels should not be used.
3. To prevent soiling the label, when pouring a liquid, the label should be uppermost.
4. For each amount to be measured, the label should be read three times
   (*a*) before removing from the cupboard,
   (*b*) before measuring the amount,
   (*c*) before replacing the container in the cupboard.
5. Only members of the pharmaceutical department are allowed to change or re-mark labels.

Rules concerning measuring:

1. Even if there is no sediment bottles of mixtures are inverted several times.
2. Only the exact amount ordered is put out.
3. Graduated measures for liquids are held at eye level and a thumbnail is placed at the height on the glass to which the medicine is to be poured. The lowest part of the meniscus is read.
4. Excess amounts, or drugs refused, are not returned to stock or put back into containers. They are thrown away.
5. The amount prepared is again checked with the prescription.

Ways of Giving Drugs. The way in which a drug is introduced into the body depends on the type of the drug, its composition, and its action. The condition of the patient is also considered.

The most simple and convenient way is by mouth. Drugs may act directly on the gastro-intestinal tract, or they may be absorbed and transferred to some remote part of the body. Drugs which are irritating to the mucous lining are generally given by some other route, but certain substances, for example cascara, are effective because they act by irritating the intestinal lining. Some drugs, such as insulin, are destroyed by gastric juice, so another route has to be selected. Other drugs are coated so that they will not dissolve until they reach the intestines.

Oral Administration. If the drug is in tablet, pill or capsule form, it should be shaken from the bottle gently into the cap, and then placed in a medicine glass or on to a spoon. Drugs should never be handled with the fingers. Water, unless contra-indicated, can be given afterwards.

Medicines that are in liquid form, and stain the teeth, can be sipped through a drinking straw.

Oily substances are better given in warmed oil measures, so that the oil will run smoothly off the porcelain. A small square of bread sprinkled with salt takes away the taste of an oil.

Nurses must not allow patients to 'help' when giving out the medicines, and patients should never be allowed to hand a medicine to another patient.

Generally ward medicine rounds are done three times or four times a day—after breakfast, after lunch and after supper, or at 10.00, 14.00, 18.00 and 22.00 hours. A trolley is set with the stock supplies of medicines, and those marked for individual patients. A variety of measures including a 5 ml spoon is required. A large water jug is needed, in case patients do not have their own water jugs. A bowl of hot soapy water and a medicine cloth are required for washing and drying the glasses. In hospital the prescriptions are written on treatment charts and are part of the patient's notes. The nurse takes the pile of these charts and the medicines are checked DIRECTLY FROM THE DOCTOR'S WRITING.

After use, bottles are wiped, containers are refitted with their lids, and they are arranged on the shelves in their usual places. Empty containers are put on one side for refilling.

Recording. Differing systems of recording drugs will be found in hospitals. The maintaining of detailed records of all drugs given, helps to prevent mistakes. Controlled Drugs are recorded in the same way. When a drug has been given, the ward register is opened at the correct page, and the date, patient's name, the time of giving, the drug and the amount of the drug are written down. The signatures of the two nurses concerned, the nurse who gave the drug, and the nurse who witnessed the measuring, the dose, and the giving, are placed in the last two columns.

Whatever system is in use, the nurses must carry out the requirements of the hospital. It is impossible to lay too much stress on the importance of checking and re-checking the amount with the prescription in order that the patient receives the correct medicament.

Dangers. Because many modern drugs resemble coloured sweets, where children are concerned, they should be placed out of sight, and beyond their reach, if possible in locked cupboards.

Tablets wrapped in foil, or in vacuum capped containers may be more difficult for a child to get at, but these handicaps are no substitute for locked cupboards.

After an illness, any tablets remaining, should be returned to the chemist, or put down a drain.

Supervision of the patient is always necessary—to see that the drug is actually swallowed—no opportunity to hoard drugs is given.

The Parenteral Administration of Drugs. When drugs are given other than by the alimentary tract, the word 'parenteral' is often used. It has come to mean the giving of a drug by a needle injection. Injection means the forcing of a fluid through a hollow tube or needle into a cavity, tissues, or a blood vessel. Drugs injected can produce a rapid action. They are not spoilt by the gastric juices. They can be given to patients who are vomiting, or who are unconscious.

Needles are to be sharp and straight if they are to be used without difficulty and without causing pain. The choice of a needle depends on the safety with which it can be used, the rate of flow of the drug to be given, the comfort of the patient, and the depth to which the needle is to penetrate. The larger the gauge number, the smaller is the diameter of the lumen. The length of needles varies. The shortest is generally suitable for a subcutaneous injection, the longest for an intramuscular injection.

Syringes. The majority are made of disposable materials. They vary in size from 1 ml. to 50 ml. They are calibrated in millimetres (or cubic centimetres) and in tenths. Syringes for vaccines and skin tests are smaller than the average syringe, and are calibrated in 1/100ths ml. An insulin syringe is calibrated in 20 marks to 1 ml.

F

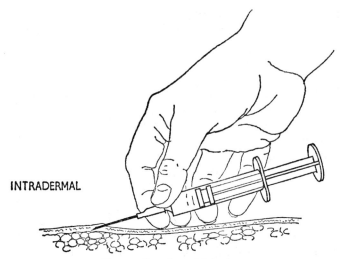

INTRADERMAL

FIG. 21 Intradermal injection

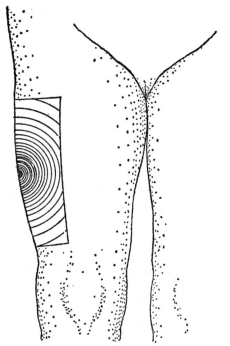

FIG. 22 Site for intramuscular injection

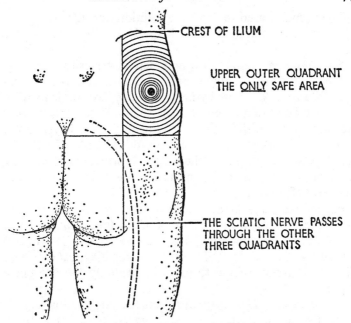

FIG. 23 Site for intramuscular injection

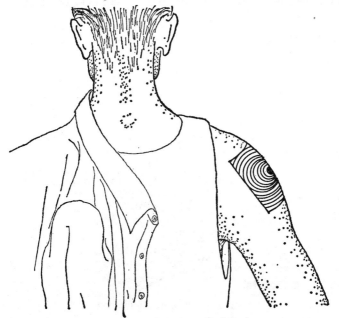

FIG. 24 Site for intramuscular injection

The plunger, used to draw the solution into the syringe, may be frosted, or coloured. This helps in reading the measured dose.

Syringes and Needles are commercially sterilised and pre-packed. They are essential for all injections. The solutions must be sterile too. After use syringes and needles are dealt with in such a way that they cannot be used again. If nurses and doctors are careless when disposing of syringes, the used syringes may find their way into the hands of drug addicts, or 'pushers', (those people who supply drugs illegally). Unprotected used needles are a potential source of danger; the points must therefore be covered before disposal.

Intradermal Injections. Because the skin contains sensory nerve endings only a small amount of a solution can be injected into the skin (intradermally) as it may be painful. This injection is used by doctors chiefly for skin tests for diagnostic purposes. The inner aspect of the forearm is generally the site chosen. Fig. 21.

Subcutaneous (*Hypodermic*) *Injections.* The drug is deposited in the tissues just beneath the skin, generally on the outer part of the arm or thigh. From 0·5 to 2 ml (cc) may be given in this

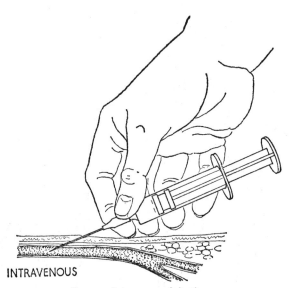

INTRAVENOUS

FIG. 25 Intravenous injection

way, and the drug will become effective in about 15 to 20 minutes. (Fig. 22).

Intramuscular Injections. When injections are to be given into muscles care must be taken to prevent the needle entering a blood vessel or nerve. The outer aspect of the thigh, or the upper outer portion of the buttock, are the areas generally chosen (see Figs. 22, 23 and 24).

Intravenous Injections. Drugs are given into a vein by a doctor and they produce an immediate effect. The veins chosen are those on the back of the hand, or the ones in the bend of the elbow (cephalic and median basilic).

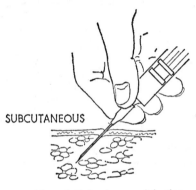

SUBCUTANEOUS

FIG. 26 Subcutaneous injection

The Giving of a Subcutaneous Injection. The skin of the area chosen is cleansed and the antiseptic allowed to dry. The drug is checked in the syringe, making sure there is no air in the syringe or needle by forcing a drop of the solution through the needle. Whilst doing this the syringe and needle are held vertically. The skin is drawn taut and the needle is inserted at a slight angle, (45 degrees) quickly, into the tissues beneath the skin, but *not* up to the hilt. The plunger is withdrawn slightly to make sure the needle is not in a blood vessel. The drug is given fairly quickly, and the area is massaged afterwards with a swab.

The Giving of an Intramuscular Injection. From 1 to 10 ml may be given in this way, and a more rapid action is produced. A large muscle is chosen, relatively free of blood vessels and nerves. The quadriceps, or the gluteal muscles are the ones most frequently used. The skin of the area is cleansed, made

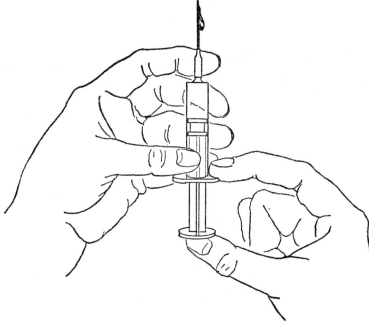

Fɪɢ. 27 Expelling air from syringe; gloves and mask may be needed if
substance being drawn up is an antibiotic.

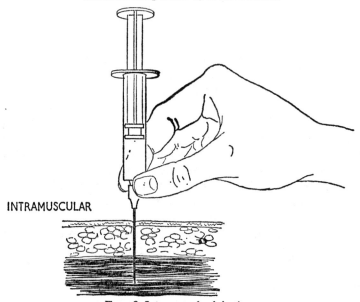

INTRAMUSCULAR

Fɪɢ. 28 Intramuscular injection

taut, and with the patient in a comfortable and relaxed position, the needle is inserted at an angle of about 90 degrees. The plunger is withdrawn a little to make sure that the needle is not in a blood vessel and the drug is injected. The area is massaged afterwards.

If a sterile syringe is not assembled ready for use, it must be handled without contaminating all the parts which must remain sterile, if the drug is to remain sterile.

If frequent injections have to be made, the site of the injection is changed.

Whenever a drug is ordered for a patient the nurse must make sure that the right amount of the right drug is given to the right patient at the right time, in the right way.

FURTHER READING

Bailey, R. E., *Pharmacology for Nurses*. Balliere, Tindall & Cassell.

Trounce, J., *Pharmacology for Nurses*. Livingstone.

CHAPTER 10

ADMINISTRATION OF OXYGEN

Air is a vital substance, taken for granted; without it no human being can live for more than five minutes. Inability to get sufficient air, or breathlessness, is a sensation which follows sudden exertion, or exercise, and everyone knows what an uncomfortable feeling it is. Some ill patients experience this symptom even when at rest, and measures must be taken to help them. If nurses are to treat their patients intelligently they must, therefore, understand the process of respiration.

Respiration is the process of supplying oxygen to the tissues and removing the waste product of carbon dioxide from the tissues. Both oxygen and carbon dioxide are carried by the blood which operates a continuous shuttle service between the lungs and the tissues. Gases are exchanged in the lungs by a process known as external respiration and this process itself consists of two parts. Inspiration is taking the air into the lungs and expiration is expelling it again, the actual air changing its composition between these two. Air is a mixture of gases; nitrogen, some rare gases found in small amounts, oxygen and carbon dioxide. The air which enters the lungs may also hold some bacteria, smoke and fumes; the amount of water vapour varies with the atmosphere and its temperature is that of the climate. Air leaving the lungs contains more carbon dioxide, less oxygen, and it is saturated with water vapour; its temperature is that of the body. The nitrogen is unchanged in human respiration and simply washes in and out of the lungs.

Mechanics of Respiration

As air is an inert substance it has to be moved in and out of the lungs and this is brought about by the movements of the respiratory muscles. These consist of the diaphragm, a thin sheet of muscle dividing the thoracic from the abdominal cavity, and the intercostal muscles, which lie between the ribs. To take in a breath, the diaphragm contracts, thus increasing the length of the thoracic cavity. The intercostal muscles also contract, pulling the ribs upwards and outwards, so increasing the width of the cavity. The lungs are then pulled out to fill this larger space and air is drawn in.

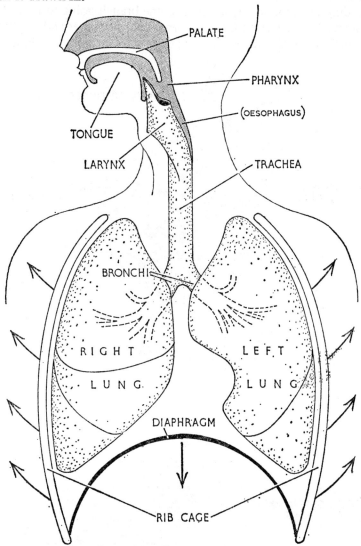

FIG. 29 The respiratory tract and movements involved in respiration

Breathing

The air enters the nose and sometimes the mouth. It is drawn into the pharynx which lies behind the nose and mouth, and from there through the larynx down into the trachea. This is a tube leading to the lungs; it bifurcates, one branch going to each of the two lungs. These tubes, or bronchi, form smaller and smaller branches and the air flows along them until it finds itself in tiny

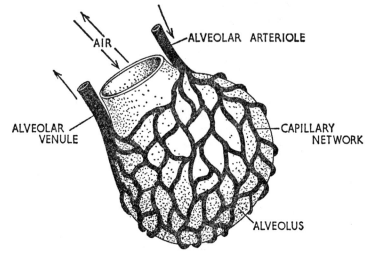

FIG. 30 An alveolus

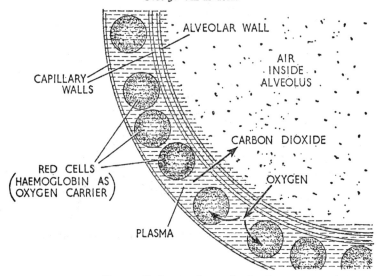

FIG. 31 Exchange of gases in alveolus

chambers or alveoli. The walls of the alveoli are very thin and circulating round them is blood, hungry for oxygen. The haemoglobin in blood takes up as much oxygen as it can. At the same time, carbon dioxide leaves the blood and enters the air in the alveoli. Having changed its composition, the air now starts on its return journey. The thoracic muscles relax, the cavity becomes smaller, the lungs retract and the air is forced out. It follows the same route as it did to come in, with the one difference that as it passes through the larynx it may be used to produce sound.

Internal Respiration

The oxygenated blood leaves the lungs in the pulmonary veins. These carry the blood to the left side of the heart and from here it is pumped to all parts of the body. Cells of all the body tissues are living things which require oxygen. They take it from the

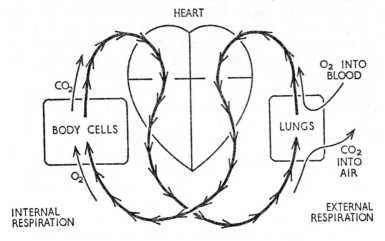

Fig. 32 Internal and external respiration

tissue fluid which has seeped through the capillary wall into the space around the cells. It passes through the cell wall into the cell. The more active the cells, the more oxygen they need. Carbon dioxide is produced and this gas is put into the blood. As this exchange takes place through the cell wall and has no communication with air, it is called internal respiration. It is, of course, the opposite of external respiration which has already taken place in the lungs.

As already mentioned, some ill patients have great difficulty with respiration; there are many causes of this symptom of dyspnoea (which simply means 'difficult breathing'). There may be some disturbances of either lungs, heart or blood; or the air itself may be altered in its composition. There may be mechanical obstruction to the free flow of air or the nervous control of respiration may fail. In each case it is logical to find and treat the cause; in many cases the treatment may include the administration of oxygen.

Supply of Oxygen

Oxygen is supplied in cylinders, which are black in colour, with white shoulders. In order to save space, the gas is compressed when the cylinder is filled, so that a large amount of oxygen can be contained within a small space. The cylinders which are actually $2\frac{1}{2}' \times 5''$ in size contain 24 cubic feet of oxygen, while the big cylinders, $4' \times 8''$, contain 120 cubic feet.

It is therefore necessary to fit a valve to the cylinder which allows the gas to escape at a reasonable rate. A gauge attached to the valve measures the amount of oxygen in the cylinder. The cylinders are opened with a key which fits the side of the valve. When the cylinder is full, oxygen often escapes with a sharp rush when the key is first turned. For this reason it is always wise to open the cylinder before connecting it to the apparatus and the patient. All nurses should make themselves familiar with the method of turning on oxygen before they have to do it by a patient's bedside, so that they may learn the knack of turning the key slowly. A flowmeter is a piece of apparatus, often incorporated with the valve, which allows control of the rate at which the gas is given to the patient. A rate of 6/8 litres per minute is usual if a face mask is used; a rather higher rate if the patient is in a tent.

Certain precautions must be strictly observed when oxygen is being used:

1. No naked light, cigarette, or mechanical toy which could spark must be allowed anywhere near the tent. Any small flame in the presence of oxygen can very easily become a serious fire which can spread with frightening rapidity if this precaution is neglected.

2. Grease must not be used on the valve or flowmeter. There is risk of an explosion occurring if this is done.

3. The cylinder must be carefully watched and not allowed to become empty. The consequences may be disastrous if the patient is enclosed within a tent and his supply of oxygen fails.

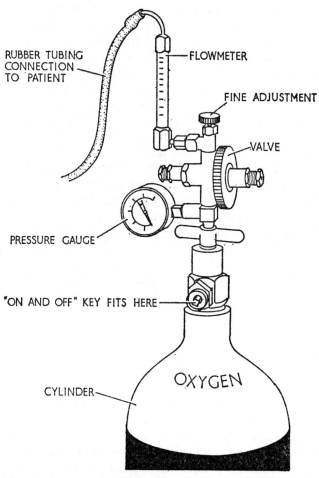

RUBBER TUBING
CONNECTION
TO PATIENT

FLOWMETER

FINE ADJUSTMENT

VALVE

PRESSURE GAUGE

"ON AND OFF" KEY FITS HERE

OXYGEN

CYLINDER

FIG. 33 Fitments to the oxygen cylinder (older type shown for clarity)

There are three ways of supplying the patient with oxygen. He may be within a tent which is kept full of the gas; he may wear a mask over his nose and mouth; or he may have small tubes introduced into his nostrils.

Oxygen Tent

An oxygen tent consists of a canopy, made of clear plastic material, which is suspended over the patient and tucked in firmly under the bedclothes. As the temperature would rise rapidly within this enclosed space, some cooling mechanism must be provided. It may consist of a large canister which is kept full of ice. As the ice melts it drains into a second canister and the first one is replenished whenever necessary. Other tents are cooled electrically. The temperature within the tent must not be allowed to exceed 21°C (70°F). A thermometer must therefore be suspended inside the tent, preferably near the patient. Openings fitted with zip fasteners allow a certain amount of attention to the patient without disturbing the whole tent. The concentration of oxygen can be maintained at a constant level and tents are invaluable for patients who cannot wear a mask. They are used for babies and young children as well as adults. In these cases a special humidifier is incorporated into the tent. Disadvantages are that the patient may feel cut off from contact with others and may get panic stricken. It is also possible to give the patient too much oxygen by this means. There may be insufficient carbon dioxide to provide the necessary stimulant for respiration and the breathing will become shallow. The patient should therefore be taken out of the tent at regular intervals.

Oxygen Masks

A number of masks have been designed for oxygen administration, but the ones in common use are made of plastic. They can be altered to fit each individual and thrown away after use. As the patient breathes out into the mask the expired air, saturated with water vapour, mixes with the oxygen coming in, and this moistens the incoming gas. Masks must fit closely if they are to be of use, and the patient who is already struggling for breath may find this almost intolerable. It is also impossible for the patient either to drink or speak whilst wearing the mask and this again may lead to further distress. It is dangerous for patients with chronic lung disease, whose respiratory centres have been damaged to use anything but a mask which limits the percentage of oxygen administered, such as a Ventimask.

Nasal Oxygen

The third method of giving oxygen is the least restricting to the patient, but the concentration of the gas cannot be maintained at a high level. Two small catheters, lubricated with an ointment containing local anaesthetic to minimise the irritation, are introduced into the nostrils. A spectacle frame is a convenient way of carrying these so that they are held out of the patient's way.

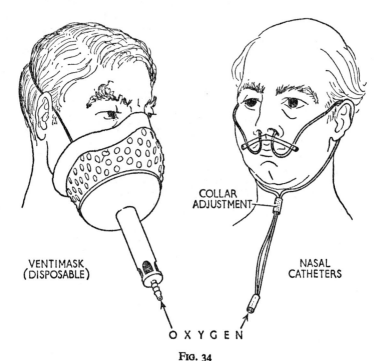

COLLAR ADJUSTMENT

VENTIMASK (DISPOSABLE)

NASAL CATHETERS

O X Y G E N

FIG. 34

(a) Disposable mask with venturi device for giving low concentration of oxygen.

(b) Nasal catheters for giving oxygen.

All patients must be carefully prepared before oxygen is given. Unfortunately they are often very ill as well as breathless and may not fully comprehend the nurse's explanation. Sometimes relatives can be of great help in this situation. The patient will often respond to the requests of a relative and he may be comforted by the presence of his wife at his bedside. Once the patient has experienced the relief gained from the treatment he will co-operate more readily.

FURTHER READING

Green, *Physiology*. Oxford.
Miller and Goode, (1960) *Man and His Body*. Gollancz.
Taverner, D., *Physiology for Nurses*. E.U.P.

CHAPTER 11

OBSERVATION AND RECORDS

When people are ill they are treated by doctors. The doctor takes a history, examines the patient, notes the signs and symptoms and then makes a diagnosis. He prescribes the treatment but leaves the nurse to carry out his orders and perform the actual bedside care.

The nurse is in a unique position because, being constantly at the bedside, she can notice at once the slightest change in the patient's condition. She can assess the reaction to treatment and, if this is unfavourable, she can inform the doctor without delay. The nurse can see clearly the course of the illness and when her observations are allied to experience she knows whether the patient is improving or deteriorating. No one can be a good nurse without being a good observer, and all nurses must cultivate this art.

General Appearance

Specific signs and symptoms are the doctor's province, but there are certain general observations which nurses make constantly. The general appearance of the patient is most important. The seriously ill patient is unable to make physical effort, so lies back on his pillows neither moving nor speaking. He does not move about in the bed, so is prone to develop pressure sores unless the nurses move him themselves. They must also give him drinks and offer urinals at appropriate intervals, for this apathetic, ill patient will not ask for these himself. Nurses should, however, talk to the patient and do all they can to encourage his hold on life. When the patient does speak or move this animation is usually a sign of improvement, and each day a little more effort can be expected.

Colour

The colour of the patient is another important feature. Certain diseases are characterized by recognizable colour changes, but the doctor who is suddenly called to see a collapsed patient will be glad to know from the nurse what the patient's colour

G

was beforehand. Pallor and flushing indicate alterations in the actual amount of blood circulating in the part, whilst cyanosis is a sign that there may be insufficient oxygen in the blood. A yellow pigmentation of the skin shows either that the body is not dealing properly with the colouring matter extracted from worn out red cells, or that bile is not passing freely into the small intestine; there are therefore a number of conditions which cause yellowing or jaundice.

Sweating

Sweating is yet another important sign, for which there are many causes. The patient may be sweating from fear, or he may be in severe pain. Some diseases, *e.g.*, thyrotoxicosis, cause the patient to sweat more than usual, whilst in other conditions a fall of body temperature may be accompanied by obvious sweating. On the other hand, the patient may simply be too hot, with too many bedclothes in a super-heated hospital ward.

Reaction to Environment

Not only physical signs should be observed. The patient's mental and emotional reaction to his environment should be noted. Patients who do not progress as well or as quickly as they might should be carefully observed, as the cause of their physical delay may well be a mental need. This can manifest itself in many ways. There may be over-dependence on the nurses, with reluctance to give up detailed nursing care. The patient may produce many apparently valid reasons why he should not get up or go home; these abnormal reactions should be both observed and dealt with. Sudden and inexplicable changes in the patient's personality are usually obvious and just as obviously require skilled treatment. Slower changes, taking place over a longer period of time may be equally important, but only the observant nurse will notice them.

Further Observations

Observations should not be confined to the senses of sight and sound. The nurse can also feel and smell. The skin of a person who is well is warm and reassuring to the touch. An ill patient may feel cold and his skin is often dry, although if he has a high temperature it will feel hot and may be moist with perspiration.

In some diseases, *e.g.*, myxoedema, the skin becomes coarse and rather harsh to the touch. The change in the texture of the skin from babyhood to old age is very striking when a woman is seen nursing her latest grandchild.

Some conditions are characterized by recognizable smells. The breath of a patient in a diabetic coma smells sweet and sickly but is quite different from the sickly smell of vomit. There may be an unpleasant smell from the pus in an abscess. Infected urine smells fishy and a chronic varicose ulcer can be detected by one's nose without ever seeing the leg.

These important observations when considered together can give an assessment of the patient and his progress. Factual data can be added to complete the picture. These facts are the body temperature, the pulse, the respiration rate, the blood pressure and the amount of fluid going into and leaving the body.

The Body Temperature

The temperature is taken with a clinical thermometer which consists of a glass bulb containing a small amount of mercury. The bulb is continuous with a calibrated glass tube up which the mercury rises as it expands with heat. The level to which it rises gives the actual temperature. The bulb of the thermometer must be inserted into the body, either into the mouth or the rectum. In Great Britain the former is commonly used with adult patients. The patient is told to hold the thermometer under his tongue and it must be left there long enough to register properly, the usual time being two minutes. The mercury will never rise to a temperature above that of the body, but it may not have time to expand properly if removed too quickly. A certain amount of practice is required to read the thermometer accurately, but once the knack has been acquired it is an easy matter. After reading the temperature the thermometer is shaken to return the mercury to the bulb.

In a small child or an unconscious patient it is neither safe nor practical to take the temperature by mouth, and the rectal method should be used. A thermometer with a short bulb of the same diameter as the stem must be used, well lubricated with Vaseline. The nurse must always hold the thermometer in position as there is some danger of it breaking if the patient should move suddenly. It is possible to place the thermometer in the axilla so that it is in contact with two skin surfaces, but it is difficult to obtain an accurate reading, and this method is seldom used. Electric thermometers are being used in many centres. The probe, covered if necessary, is inserted into the mouth, axilla or rectum.

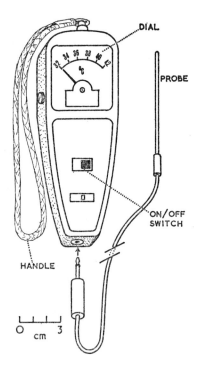

Electric Thermometer

The normal body temperature of an adult is fairly constant between 36°–37°C (97°–99°F). A rise above this usually indicates either infection or damage to the heat regulating centre in the brain. A fall below 36°C is seen when the patient is shocked or in a state of collapse. It may also be seen in very cold weather, when babies and old people have difficulty in maintaining their body temperature. If the heating is inadequate or the room cold, the body temperature falls and the person suffers from hypothermia. The condition is a serious one and can cause death if untreated. In the winter health visitors carry special low reading thermometers so that they can check the temperature of a baby or an old person who seems cold and lethargic.

The temperature may be taken twice daily or more frequently. A record is kept on a chart and it is important to mark the chart immediately after reading the thermometer.

The Pulse

The patient's pulse is usually taken at the same time as the temperature. It is the rhythmic throb of the arteries as the heart pumps the blood round. The pulse is therefore an indication of the state of the heart and circulation. All the arteries in the body pulsate, but it is only the ones which run near the surface which can be felt. The most convenient of these is the radial artery which can be felt on the thumb side of the wrist. Slight pressure of the nurse's fingers over the artery enables her to feel the pulsations and they can easily be counted. The rate is expressed in beats per minute, so a watch with a seconds hand is essential to time the beats. The pulse rate in a baby is about 140 beats per minute. During childhood this rate gradually falls until the adult rate of 70–80 is reached. Wide variations of this rate are seen in illness, nearly all of them being more rapid than usual. Slower pulse rates are far less common. There are many causes for an increased pulse rate; the most usual being excitement, fear, exertion, infection, shock and haemorrhage. The pulse rate is recorded on the same chart as the temperature and, again, should be written down immediately it has been counted. In addition to the rate of the pulse, its rhythm and strength should be observed. Alterations in rhythm clearly indicate that the heart is not pumping regularly and this may be a serious sign. The strength of the pulse is related to the state of the heart muscle and the total volume of circulating blood. Much valuable information is gained from careful observation of the pulse.

The Respirations

The third recording on the chart is that of the respiration rate, this again being counted per minute. As respiration can be partly controlled by the will it is impossible to get an accurate record of this rate if a conscious patient is aware that it is being observed. The respiration rate should therefore be counted either during sleep or when the patient's attention is diverted. In actual fact little attention is paid to the actual rate of respiration. A far more important observation is the type of respiration, and whether or not the patient has difficulty in breathing. This latter symptom, called dyspnoea, is an important one and denotes disease of either heart or lungs. The character of the breathing changes in illness and may become noisy or deeper than usual. The patient who has had a sudden loss of blood will be starving for oxygen and draw in great gasping breaths. If he is also restless, further bleeding should be suspected, and this is an instance of where prompt response to observation may save the patient's life.

The Blood Pressure

All pumps which move fluid must exert pressure to do so. The heart is no exception. The force behind each beat of the heart can be measured and recorded in the blood pressure. To do this an instrument called a sphygmomanometer is used. (An awkward word; sphygmus is from the Greek and means pulse; a manometer is an instrument which measures pressure.) The cuff of the sphygmomanometer is applied to the upper arm and air is pumped into it. It is attached by rubber tubing to a column of mercury which will record the actual pressure in millimetres. Air in the cuff presses on the arm and when the pressure within it is a little higher than the pressure within the brachial artery the sound of the pulsating artery cannot be heard when a stethoscope is applied over the artery at the elbow. Air is slowly let out of the cuff and the pressure falls; when the two pressures equalise, the throbbing of the artery can be heard again. This moment of equalization of pressure occurs when the heart is contracting and therefore showing the greater force. As the contraction of the heart is known as the systole, the reading of the mercury gives the systolic pressure. When the pressure within the sphygmomanometer cuff is at its lowest level, the sound changes its character and this is the diastolic pressure. The heart is now in its phase of relaxation. The procedure of taking blood pressure is essentially one which must be learnt by practical experience. It is recorded on the appropriate chart.

Points to Note

Nurses should remember, however, that when the cuff is dilated to a pressure above that of the patient's blood pressure the arterial supply to the arm is cut off. The patient will experience severe pain if this is not released fairly quickly. It is also important to ensure that the patient is relaxed and comfortable. The arm should be taken out of the sleeve so that it does not constrict the blood supply. The sphygmomanometer should be on a firm base sufficiently near the bed to ensure no tension on the rubber tubing. Nurse should also be comfortable and in a position from which she can easily see the column of mercury. Although blood pressure may be a useful piece of information to know, it must be emphasized that much practice is essential before anyone can make an accurate reading.

The last factual observation is the record of fluid taken into the body and that last from the body. This intake and output chart is a valuable assessment in certain specified conditions and has been described in chapter 8.

Reports

To be of any value, all these observations must be used. They form the basis of reports, both oral and written, which nurses give to one another. This information is then passed on to the doctor when he visits the patient.

Charts are continued by whoever makes the observation so that a continuous record of temperature, pulse, respirations, intake and output and, if necessary, blood pressure, is available at any time.

Oral reports on the patient are given from one nurse when she is relieved by another. In every case the nurse receiving the report must be absolutely certain that she has entirely understood what she has been told. Mistakes or omissions may have very serious consequences. Some words can easily be muddled when spoken—oral and aural, for instance, are pronounced alike. Written reports are much safer and should be used whenever possible. They are made on a card which is kept for the patient in a *Kardex* folder or possibly in a book which covers all the ward patients.

The report should give a picture of the patient during the time covered by the report. His general condition should be noted and attention drawn to any obvious sign or symptom. Any complaints the patient may have made should be noted. Operations or treatments should be detailed. All Controlled Drugs given must be reported and other drugs, if these are in any way different from previous medication. Any instructions or requests should be at the end of the report. In hospital it is usual to report in detail on all new patients, any patient who has had an operation and all seriously ill people. Patients who have improved so that they are convalescent do not have such detailed reports as there is little to notify. Reports should always be written with care and details verified. They are not only the records of daily and nightly observations on the patient, but are used to provide continuity of nursing care and treatment. They may be of extreme importance much later, especially if doubts or queries arise and it becomes essential to check the full details of the patient's progress. They must be written legibly, in ink, and finally signed with a recognizable signature.

CHAPTER 12

THE SANITARY NEEDS OF
THE PATIENT (1)

The healthy person, completely orientated in society and occupied with work, pays little attention to the processes of elimination, which become part of daily routine, controlled by the habit pattern of the individual. When there is a break in the normal habit pattern, due to change of environment, or illness, attention may be drawn to the elimination of the body's waste products.

When a person becomes a hospital patient it may appear that the passing of urine and faeces—waste products from the kidneys and large intestine—is a matter of great importance. The patient may wonder why questions have to be asked by the nurse, and although the nurse does this as part of her duty, she must realise that it can be very embarrassing for the patient.

The unconscious patient cannot answer questions and the nurse must observe the patient for herself. Urine may be retained in the bladder, and the patient's abdomen becomes distended. On the other hand the patient may pass urine involuntarily.

Elimination from the Kidneys

There are two kidneys situated in the middle of the back, one on either side of the vertebral column. Blood passes through the kidneys and unwanted water and substances such as urea are extracted from it. This water, and the waste products it contains, is called urine. Some of these waste products are formed in the body as the cells carry out their different functions, others are from the diet which is taken into the body. Urine is being manufactured all the time, the actual rate of production being approximately one millilitre a minute. As it is obviously impractical for urine to leave the body the whole time, urine is stored until a reasonable quantity has accumulated. The storage reservoir is a membranous bag called the bladder which is situated in the pelvis. Urine from the kidneys drips down two

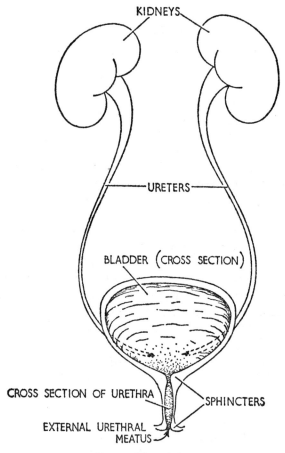

FIG. 35 The urinary tract

tubes, called the ureters, and gradually the bladder fills. Another tube connects the bladder with the external body surface; this outlet tube is the urethra.

Emptying the Bladder

When the amount of urine is large enough, the bladder walls begin to stretch and the nervous system is involved. This system is the communication system of the body and conveys the message that the bladder is full and must be emptied. What happens next is dependent on the age and state of health of the person involved. In a small baby, the bladder is emptied as soon as the message is received; this is known as reflex action, and the baby has a wet napkin. In a young child there will be a certain amount of control and as long as the child's patience is not taxed too strongly the bladder will be emptied when the child reaches his 'potty'. With adult life there comes increasing control of activity so that adults only pass urine, or micturate, as it is called, when it is socially convenient to do so.

In illness, however, this control may break down. The liaison between the bladder and brain may be faulty or even severed altogether. There may be actual disease of the urinary tract. The person may be unconscious and be oblivious to the communications brought to his brain. It is interesting to note, however, that one of the causes of restlessness in an unconscious patient is a full bladder. The good nurse can often prevent a wet bed by observing this restlessness and putting a bedpan or urinal in place.

Patients' Problems

When some patients are confined to bed they may find difficulties when they try to use a bedpan or urinal. An understanding nurse will always see that a patient is given an opportunity to respond promptly to the desire to pass urine. If it is not contrary to the treatment, she will also see that the patient has plenty of fluids to drink to assist the normal excretion of urine.

There are times when the bladder is filled with urine, and the patient has the desire to pass it, but he just cannot. There are several things a nurse can do. With the patient in position on a bedpan, or with a urinal, the sound of running water may help. Warm water poured over the vulva, increasing the intake of water or fruit juice, or just allowing the patient to stand out of bed, are other means which can be tried. If the patient cannot stand out of bed, the bedpan can be placed along the edge of the bed, and with the patient's feet supported on a chair, a more natural position is assumed.

Even though absolute privacy is ensured, some patients are tense and anxious if a nurse is around. It is better, in these circumstances, for the nurse to leave the patient, if he will come to no harm.

Difficulties in passing urine whilst confined to bed might be summarized as follows:

(*a*) apprehension at being in hospital
(*b*) lack of familiarity with the bedpan and the way to use it
(*c*) lack of privacy, and
(*d*) the unnatural position in bed.

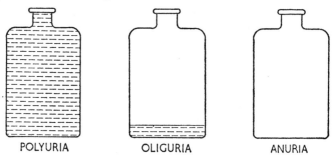

POLYURIA   OLIGURIA   ANURIA

Fig. 36 Differences in urinary output

Responsibilities of the Nurse

It is the nurse's responsibility to inform the sister of the ward if the patient is not passing sufficient urine, or if there is a gross difference between the fluid intake and the urinary output.

As a nurse in training gains experience she will know that in the disease of diabetes mellitus an unusually large amount of urine is excreted (polyuria). In certain heart diseases, when the circulation is impaired, the output of urine may be decreased (oliguria). In acute kidney failure there may be no urine at all (anuria).

When the kidneys are working normally the patient may need to pass urine four hourly, or six hourly, during the day. From about 200 to 300 ml are passed at a time. A bedpan or urinal is offered to a patient on waking and opportunities must be provided during the day, and again at night just before the patient is made comfortable and is ready to sleep.

The volume of urine passed is noted when a fluid balance chart is being recorded for the patient.

Elimination from the Large Intestine

The solid waste material excreted from the large intestine is known as faeces. When the small intestine has dealt with the

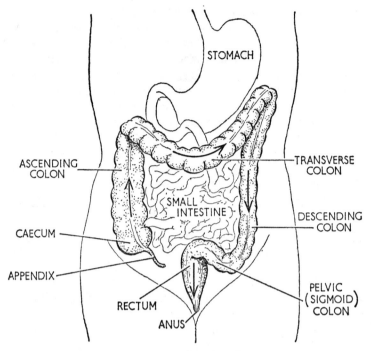

FIG. 37 The large intestine

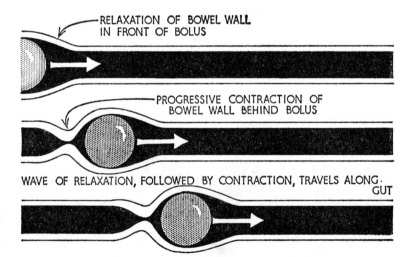

FIG. 38 Peristalsis

great work of digestion and absorption, waste material passes into the large intestine. This residue is of little value. It contains material that cannot be digested, such as the cellulose stalks of green leaves, skins of fruits, and seeds. Dead cells, salts, pigment and mucus are also in this residue. If drugs taken by mouth are not completely absorbed small quantities will be excreted too. In the small intestine bacteria decompose carbohydrates to acid and gas. Some of these bacteria pass into the large intestine and help to form the faeces. They also help to make vitamins B and K which, with water and salts, are absorbed into the blood vessels of the intestinal walls. As the water is absorbed the semi-solid mass which is left passes by peristaltic action and gradually accumulates in the distal part of the colon. Peristalsis is a muscular movement by which contents of a tube are propelled onwards. According to the habit of the individual peristalsis may be set in motion by the intake of food.

Emptying the Bowels

Normally the rectum is empty, or almost empty, and the anal opening is closed by the contraction of the internal and the external ring (sphincter) muscles. Through peristaltic action faecal material enters the rectum. Sensory nerve endings are stimulated and the desire for defaecation is produced. Defaecation is the expelling of faeces from the rectum by powerful

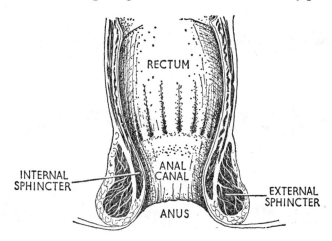

FIG. 39 Internal and external sphincters

peristalsis of the colon. Voluntary contraction of the abdominal muscles, pelvic floor and diaphragm help to empty the rectum. Intestinal gas is excreted with the faeces.

Failure to respond to this call of nature results in constipation. Faeces are retained in the rectum as there is no return mechanism. They lose water, become dry, hard and more difficult to expel.

In the infant, when a mass peristaltic movement causes the contents of the distal colon to enter the rectum, the act of defaecation occurs immediately. The anal sphincters relax, the rectum shortens and the muscles contract. The pressure inside the abdomen is so great that the venous circulation is impeded and the child appears 'red in the face'. Later in life, social convention requires that defaecation be controlled, and training establishes a habit time.

Bowel Habits

The majority of people have a normal daily bowel habit, but in a number of healthy and perfectly fit persons the bowels may be opened from once a week to four times a day. There is a wide range of normality. The only ill effects of constipation are discomfort and faecal impaction, but for many generations a fear has existed connecting internal poisons with constipation. The bowels, like cesspools and sewers, were thought to require constant clearings. Many people participate in artificial purging even today. Constant use of laxatives and liquid paraffin is known to be harmful. They cause fatigue of the colon, and interfere with the absorption of vitamins.

Safe Disposal of Excreta

Safe disposal of excreta is essential, as infection is carried in it. Bacterial diseases of the alimentary tract add harmful microorganisms, and there may be ova from intestinal worms. Lavatory pans have a water seal in the bend of the discharge pipe to prevent unpleasant air entering the building. The water carriage system allows faeces and urine to pass quickly into sloping drains and sewers far below the streets of the town.

There were few sewers in Great Britain until the nineteenth century. Sewage drained into the local river, or into a barrel put into the back yard of the house. In this way cholera and typhoid fever were spread very easily as drinking water was drawn direct from the rivers.

Today, sewage is efficiently treated and rendered harmless in modern sewage works. The solid particles are separated from the fluid and this sludge is dumped far out at sea by special tankers, or used to make manure. The purified fluid is run into the rivers. In country districts cruder methods are used.

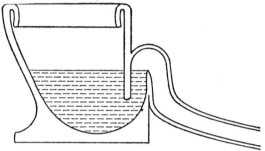

FIG. 40 Lavatory pan with water seal

Factors which Interfere with Normal Elimination

Some common causes of constipation are:
1. Neglect in answering the 'call of nature'—bad habit formation.
2. Lack of exercise—resulting in decreased peristaltic action.
3. A low residue diet with very little roughage—so there is insufficient bulk to form the faeces.
4. Insufficient fluid intake—causing dry, hard faeces.
5. Confinement to bed—causing an unnatural position for defaecation.
6. Depression.
7. Pressure—a growth in the pelvis.
8. Handling of the intestines during abdominal operations.

Means of Overcoming Constipation

Natural means of overcoming constipation are:
(a) Establishment of a good bowel habit—a regular time each day.
(b) Muscular exercise.
(c) A diet which contains brown bread, fresh vegetables, fresh fruit or prunes which assist the body's natural actions.
(d) Drinking large quantities of fluid.

The patient to-day is subjected to a barrage of advertisements when drugs and proprietary substances are recommended in an effort to overcome constipation. Great claims are made by manufacturers, but nothing is said about the fact that continued use considerably hinders the functioning of the large intestine.

Patients' Problems

Whenever the condition allows, and the doctor has given permission, patients are encouraged to get out of bed and they are assisted to the lavatory. The dressing gown and nightwear are arranged comfortably, and the patient helped and lowered on to the lavatory seat. The nurse should stay within calling distance, and be prepared to help the patient off the seat, giving whatever assistance may be required.

Use of Lavatory Chair or 'Sanichair'

The lavatory chair is a chair on wheels, but the seat is shaped like a lavatory seat. It can be used in two ways. A bedpan can be placed under the seat, and the chair then acts as a commode. If preferred a patient can be wheeled to the lavatory. The chair is placed in position over the seat of the lavatory, and the patient then has 'up-patient' facilities without having to walk at all.

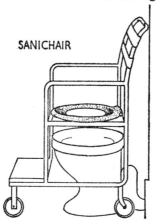

FIG. 41 Sanichair

Use of Commode

A commode can be used for patients who find trying to balance on a bedpan too much of an effort. This is especially applicable

H

to patients with certain cardiac (heart) conditions. A commode is a kind of chair with a container for excreta fitted into the seat, covered with a lid. The chair is made of unpolished wood or

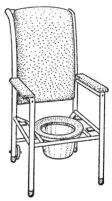

FIG. 42 Commode (seat cover not shown)

metal so that it can be washed and scrubbed. When placed by the bed, the patient can be lifted out on to the commode so the strain of using a bedpan is lessened. Afterwards the removable container can be lifted out, emptied, washed and refitted very easily.

The Giving of a Bedpan

Unfortunately there are some patients who must stay in bed. The satisfactory use of a bedpan is no easy task. It requires almost an acrobatic feat for some patients.

Screens are drawn round the patient and the nurse should make sure that there is nothing to inhibit the desire to defaecate or pass urine. He is placed on the bedpan in the position that is most comfortable for him.

The bedpan is warmed to a comfortable temperature in the sluice room and carried, covered, preferably with a disposable paper cover, to the patient. It is a fairly simple procedure to give a bedpan to a patient in the recumbent position. The nurse should first make certain that the patient's nightwear is clear of the bedpan. Standing by the bed the nurse loosens and lifts the top bedclothes. Making sure that the patient's nightwear is clear, she places the bedpan on the bed beside the patient. The open, deeper end of the bedpan should be towards the foot of the bed, and the side of the bedpan parallel to the side of the bed. With her left hand under the small of the patient's back (the nurse being at the right hand side of the patient's bed) the nurse can raise the patient's buttocks. The patient is instructed to bend his knees and press his feet firmly on the bed. As the patient 'lifts', the bedpan is carefully placed under the buttocks, the nurse moving it into position with her right hand. This can be done with little exposure of the patient.

With the bedpan in position the nurse makes sure that the patient is comfortable and supported. If he is able to care for himself, a roll of toilet paper is put within easy reach. If the patient is weak and ill and cannot co-operate as easily as he might wish, another nurse is needed to help in lifting him, and adjusting the bedpan to the proper position.

Unless it is contraindicated the patient should be left on his own, to use the bedpan in privacy, but the nurse should never be far away. If it is essential that the nurse must remain in the room, or behind the screens, she can help to make the situation less embarrassing if she busily engages in some other activity, like tidying the locker, for instance. This will allow her to watch the patient carefully, without seeming to do so.

The Removing of a Bedpan

The patient is again instructed to press his feet firmly on the bed and help by bending his knees and raising his buttocks from the bedpan. The nurse grasps the side of the bedpan firmly with her right hand, using her left to support the patient. The bedpan is moved to the side and the patient lowered on to the bed. (Inexperienced nurses need to be reminded that the bedpan should not be grasped by the fingers curving around the upper edge. It is not necessary to touch the inside of the bedpan at all, and if the nurse does, she will contaminate her hand). After use the bedpan must be carefully moved, otherwise the contents may be spilt.

The Care of the Patient

Patients who are able to care for themselves will want to do so, but the nurse will have to provide a bowl of warm water, and the necessary articles for the patient to wash and dry his hands thoroughly.

Very ill patients, or patients unable to care for themselves, will require the services of a nurse. They may be embarrassed because someone else has to care for them, after the use of a bedpan, but the nurse can relieve the patient of unnecessary embarrassment by her actions and manner. Careful draping of the patient, avoiding exposure, and an attitude that she is there to be of service in just such a situation, will help considerably.

When removing the bedpan the patient is turned immediately on to his left side. The anal area is cleansed with toilet paper, or special tissues, and if necessary, the buttocks are washed with soap and water.

The Giving of a Urinal

Whereas female patients use bedpans for passing urine, and/or faeces, the male patients use urinals for the voiding of urine, and bedpans for faeces. When a male patient asks for a bedpan, a urinal must be given to him as well.

On admission it must be explained to a male patient, if he is to be confined to bed, that the word 'urinal' is used, and its purpose mentioned. The word 'bottle' is frequently used by male patients. New patients may not know what to ask for when they want to pass urine. If this information is not given to them, it may result in the discomfort of bladder distension.

Many patients are able to place a urinal in position without assistance. The nurse need only carry it, covered, to the patient's bed, and hand it to the patient.

If the patient is unable to use the urinal without assistance, a nurse must place it in position, in such a way that the contents will not be spilt. Screens are drawn and the top bedclothes are moved, and the patients nightwear arranged so that he is not needlessly exposed. The legs need to be slightly apart, so that the urinal can be on the bed between them. With the nurse at the right hand side of the bed, the urinal is held in her right hand, close to the scrotum. With the left hand the penis is directed into the opening. The urinal is held so that the urine will not flow backwards, and out into the bed.

The Removing of a Urinal

The urinal is removed by withdrawing it carefully from in between the patient's legs. The opening must be directed upwards so that urine is not spilt.

The patient who can help himself will remove it from beneath the bedclothes, hand it to the nurse, and she will cover it and take it away. Many beds have containers fitted to the long rails of the bedstead for holding urinals. Nurses need to be alert to their presence, remember to empty them when necessary, and not knock them when bedmaking.

Female Urinals

Specially constructed urinals are sometimes used for female patients, especially orthopaedic patients, if they find difficulty in using a bedpan. An example is the 'Stanmore' pattern.

Emptying Bedpans and Urinals

Bedpans and urinals are carried to a sluice room for emptying. Bedpans may be put into bedpan washers, when, on closing the doors, the contents are emptied and the bedpans are washed thoroughly. They may be sterilized. The contents pass into the main sewerage system of the hospital.

If there are no bedpan washers, the contents are emptied into a 'hopper', a kind of lavatory pan. Urinals are also emptied into this, and after emptying, they are washed thoroughly by the nurse. Rinsing the bedpan in cold water helps to prevent coagulation of protein material in the waste products. Brushes are frequently kept for the purpose, in containers with disinfectant, and are to be used in the cleaning process. Faecal material tends to lodge under the rim of the bedpan. Many hospitals have bedpan washer/sterilisers in the sanitary annexes; others have large tank-like boilers for the same purpose.

Disposable bedpans and urinals are available in some hospitals. After use they are placed in a commercial container where they are reduced to a fine pulp suitable for draining into the sewerage system.

Containers for measuring urine are kept in the sluice rooms, and the nurse should not dispose of the urine if she is in any doubt as to whether or not the patient's fluid balance is being recorded.

The nurse must never fail to wash her hands thoroughly when this service has been carried out for the patient.

FURTHER READING

Norton, Exton, Smith & McLaren, *An Investigation on Geriatric Nursing Problems in Hospital.* National Association for the Care of Old People.

Rudd, *The Nursing of the Elderly Sick.* Faber.

Taverner, (1961) *Physiology for Nurses.* E.U.P.

CHAPTER 13

THE SANITARY NEEDS OF
THE PATIENT (2)

Disturbances of Micturition

Disturbances of micturition are common and nurses spend a fair amount of time dealing with them. RETENTION is the term used to describe a full bladder which the patient cannot empty unaided, and there are many causes of this. If the bladder is so full that it simply cannot stretch to hold another drop, then the urine will dribble out at the same rate as the kidneys are putting it in. This uncomfortable state of affairs is known as RETENTION WITH OVERFLOW. If control of micturition is lost, the bladder will empty when it is full. This reversal to babyhood is called INCONTINENCE.

In many of these cases it is necessary to drain urine out of the bladder by some artificial means. This procedure is called catheterization. A catheter is a hollow tube which has a smooth tip in which there is a side opening. The catheter is passed up the urethra and when the tip reaches the bladder, urine flows out of the other end. The technique of catheterization varies with the sex of the patient.

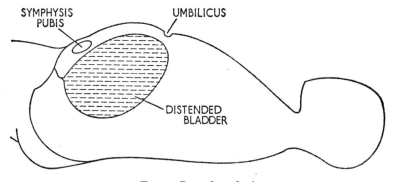

FIG. 43 Retention of urine

Catheterization of a Woman

In the pelvis of a woman there are three organs which open on to the external surface of the body. The rectum is at the back and

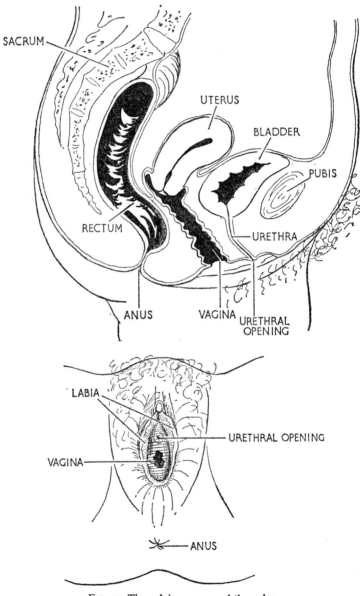

FIG. 44 The pelvic organs and the vulva

Its opening is the back passage or anus. In the middle lies the womb or uterus with the vaginal opening, and in front of this is the urethral opening leading to the bladder. The urethra is about five centimetres long, so it is a comparatively easy matter to guide the catheter up to the bladder.

Preparation of the Apparatus

This is dealt with first. As there is a risk that infection might be introduced into the bladder during this procedure it is carried out with aseptic precautions.

Equipment needed:

(a) A Sterile Pack Containing:	(b) Other Requirements:
2 dressing towels	Bottle of warm sterile lotion
1 kidney dish	Lubricant, if used
2 catheters (size 8)	Sterile specimen jars, if required
1 small bowl	Paper bag for used swabs
10 cotton wool swabs	Paper bag for used instruments
2 pairs forceps.	Lamp.

Preparation of the Patient

The patient is prepared by drawing the curtains to ensure privacy and giving her an explanation of what is about to happen. She will naturally be somewhat apprehensive, but she can be reassured that although she will feel the catheter entering, it will not cause pain. The patient lies on her back with a pillow for her head, and she is asked to bend her knees and let her legs fall apart. This position allows the nurse to have the best possible view of the area, but at the same time it gives the patient the maximum amount of embarrassment. Sympathy and kindness allied to an explanation of why this is necessary will overcome the patient's shyness and she will be assured that the procedure will not take long. The bedclothes are turned back to the knees and a good light, such as an anglepoise lamp, is arranged in position.

The Technique

The nurse washes and dries her hands thoroughly before touching any apparatus. The pack is opened on the trolley which is placed within reach. The nurse washes her hands again. Towels are placed around the vulval region. The kidney dish is put between the legs to receive the urine. The area is carefully swabbed to remove surface contamination. To reduce the risk of infection, the swabs are wiped down the area from above and are discarded after each wipe. Separation of the labia with the left hand allows the nurse to have a good view and the opening of the urethra can be seen above the vagina. Using forceps, the eye of the catheter is gently inserted into the urethra. As soon as the eye is in the bladder urine will flow out of the end of the catheter into the kidney dish. When the bladder is empty the catheter is withdrawn and the patient swabbed dry, remembering to dry the cleft of the patient's buttocks. The bedclothes are replaced and the patient is left comfortable.

Catheterization of a Man

In men the urinary system is intimately connected with the reproductive system and is in fact referred to as the genito-urinary system. The urethra is enclosed within the penis and is approximately eighteen centimetres long; as it leaves the bladder it passes through the prostate gland. Enlargement or growth of this gland therefore leads to obstruction of the urethra with consequent retention of urine, a fairly common condition among middle-aged and elderly men. The male urethra may also be the site of inflammation which in turn may lead to narrowing or stricture.

Catheterization of a man is therefore rather more difficult. Not only is the urethra much longer, but there may be actual mechanical obstruction within it. The procedure is carried out by a doctor or a male nurse; in the former instance the nurse is required to prepare the apparatus.

Types of Catheters

There are many different patterns of catheters, and they are made of either plastic or rubber; the former are now more commonly used. In many cases the catheter is left in position in the bladder so a self-retaining pattern must be used. Illustrated are two patterns, Foley's and Malecot's. A Malecot's catheter needs an introducer, and a Foley's catheter has a balloon which has to be filled with either sterile water or air.

In addition to the requirements for a female catheterization the following are necessary:

A sterile lubricant, such as KY jelly, or xylocaine gel,
1 20 ml. syringe, for Foley's catheter only,
1 clip or spiggot for end of catheter.

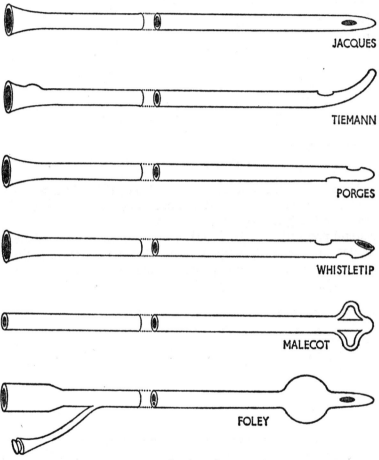

FIG. 45 Types of catheter in common use

A self-retaining catheter may either drain continuously
through sterile tubing into a plastic bag or bottle by the side of
the bed, or it may be clipped off and the bladder drained at
intervals.

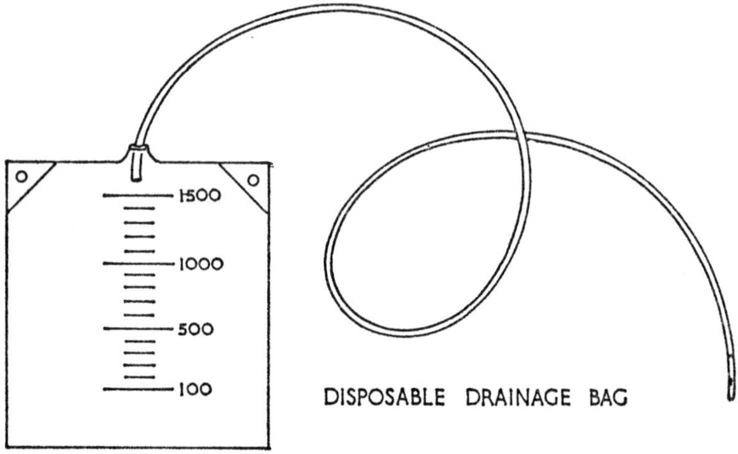

1500

1000

500

100

DISPOSABLE DRAINAGE BAG

FIG. 46 Disposable drainage bag

Whenever catheterization is carried out, either in a man or a woman, it must be stressed that in every case there is a risk of infection being carried up the urethra to the bladder. The most careful precautions must be taken to avoid this. Most catheters to-day are supplied ready for use. They have been sterilized during the manufacturing process, often by exposure to radiation, and then sealed in plastic bags. The catheter is removed

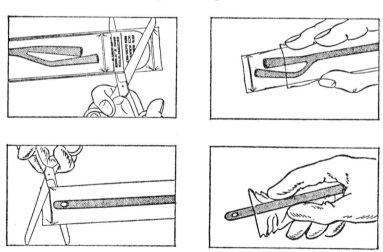

FIG. 47 Use of pre-sterilized packaged catheter

from the outer bag at the beginning of the procedure, then only released from the inner one immediately before it is introduced into the bladder. The inner bag is snipped at the end and then it can be used to cover the catheter so that the latter is never touched by either hands or forceps. The catheter is thrown away after use. Non disposable catheters must be sterilized with care in an autoclave before being used.

The procedure must never be carried out unless it is absolutely necessary; the three main reasons for it being:

(a) to relieve retention,

(b) to ensure an empty bladder before any operation and procedure in its vicinity, or

(c) to obtain a sterile specimen of urine.

Incontinence

Involuntary excretion of urine and faeces may occur in patients who are very young, very old, very ill or unconscious. It may also occur in times of stress—perhaps on admission to hospital, due to the strange environment. After operations on the urinary tract the patient may find it difficult to control micturition. Similarly if there is severe diarrhoea, it is not easy for the patient to control the anal sphincter and remain clean. In every case of incontinence, the cause should be sought and treated where possible.

Care of the Incontinent Patient

The patient who is incontinent requires careful nursing to keep him clean and comfortable and free from pressure sores. Use should be made of the fact that the bladder and bowel can be trained to empty at certain times. At regular intervals, say every three hours, the patient should be taken to the lavatory, or sat on a commode or given a bedpan or urinal. With perseverance and patience a regular routine is established and a wet or dirty bed becomes the exception rather than the rule.

Patients must never be left wet or dirty. The soiled clothes should be removed at once and the skin thoroughly washed and carefully dried. A waterproofing cream or silicone spray may then be applied and the patients position changed. Incontinence pads, pads made of cellulose wadding and paper, are useful to save laundry, they must be removed and fresh ones replaced as soon as they are wet.

Involuntary excretion is very distressing for the conscious patient. A good nurse will not show by any action or words that the duties of attending to him are unpleasant in any way, neither will she 'scold' him for not having sufficient control.

It may be a help for her to remember that her attitude when attending to the patient's sanitary needs influences the patient's attitudes towards these essential functions.

Abdominal Discomfort

When a patient is confined to bed at home, or in hospital, normal habits are interfered with and faeces may be retained. Flatus (intestinal gas) is not passed either, and this gas accumulates in the intestines giving rise to discomfort, abdominal distension, and later, pain.

To relieve a patient in this condition a flatus tube can be lubricated and inserted through the anal opening into the rectum, for about ten centimetres. It is advisable to place the other end under water in a bowl. The rising of bubbles indicates the passage of flatus.

Faecal Impaction

If constipation is present for a long time, faeces accumulate in the rectum and become hard and impacted. A small amount of liquid material may escape from the anus at intervals, a condition known as spurious diarrhoea. Medical examination will confirm the diagnosis and then the impacted faeces must be removed by hand. A rubber glove is worn, the index finger well lubricated and inserted into the rectum. Without causing discomfort to the patient the mass is broken up into small parts. By extracting the broken sections the entire mass which blocked the rectum may be removed fairly easily; further treatment may be necessary to clear up this condition completely and establish normal function.

Rectal Suppositories

Rectal suppositories are cone-shaped, and made of a variety of substances depending on the purpose for which they are to be used. They are commonly used to promote evacuation of faeces, as they cause little discomfort to the patient. At ordinary room temperature they retain their shape, but melt when subjected to body heat in the rectum.

Soap or glycerine suppositories are used to expel faeces. Irritation by the suppository stimulates the rectum to expel its

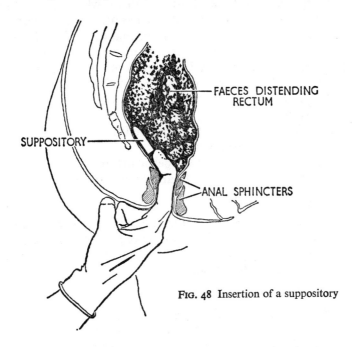

FAECES DISTENDING RECTUM

SUPPOSITORY

ANAL SPHINCTERS

FIG. 48 Insertion of a suppository

entire contents, including the suppository itself. The hygroscopic action of glycerine increases the bulk, which has a further irritating effect. Excellent results can be obtained by the use of proprietary suppositories. *Dulcolax* is one which works when in contact with the mucous lining of the rectum.

For inserting a suppository, a rubber glove, or a finger stall with a cape should be worn. The paper covering is removed and the suppository is dipped in hot water. It is passed into the rectum until the sphincters grip on the second joint of the nurse's finger. After insertion pressure should be applied over the anus for a few moments until the desire to expel the suppository is over. The patient is left comfortable, encouraged to retain the suppository for as long as possible, but told to ask for a bedpan when one is required. The nurse makes sure that the bowel action has been satisfactory.

Enemas

Although constipation can be avoided by diet, and the use of suppositories brings relief to a patient who is unfortunate enough to become constipated, enemas are sometimes ordered. The term 'enema' is defined as 'an injection of fluid into the rectum and lower bowel'. There are many types of enemas, but the type commonly used is the cleansing enema. It removes faeces from the rectum and lower bowel. It may be given when normal evacuation does not seem possible.

It may be used:
(*a*) before operation on the intestinal tract
(*b*) before X-ray examination
(*c*) before examination of the pelvic organs, or
(*d*) before fluid which is to be absorbed is given rectally.

Disposable Enemas

These are supplied ready for use and full instructions are printed on the packet. They consist of a plastic bag containing the fluid (usually sodium phosphate or dioctyl and glycerine) with a rectal nozzle attached.

Preparation of the Apparatus

Equipment needed: The enema
Lubricant, e.g. vaseline
Linen or paper squares
Paper towel
Bedpan (or commode)

Preparation of the Patient

Having made certain that the patient understands the procedure, is in no draught, and that his privacy is ensured, one pillow is left under the head, and the patient turned into the left lateral position, with knees drawn up. The bedclothes are turned back, but the patient is not exposed. The buttocks are placed on a paper towel along the edge of the bed. The upper leg is placed over the lower leg. (If this position is not possible, the enema may be given with the patient lying on his back). A urinal is offered to a male patient.

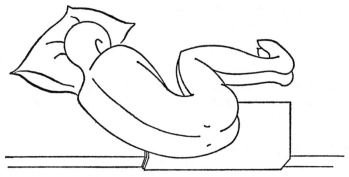

FIG. 49 Left lateral position (upper bedclothes not shown)

The Technique

The tip of the nozzle of the enema is removed and the nozzle is lubricated with vaseline. It is then inserted into the rectum for 8–10 cms and the bag is gently squeezed, so injecting the contents into the rectum. The nozzle is then withdrawn and the patient is encouraged to retain the enema for a short time before being given a bedpan.

It is left to the nurse to decide whether or not to stay with the patient. If the patient is light-headed, or distressed, or ill, she should remain with him. In any case she should be within call. Any flatus passed should be noted.

When the patient has finished, the bedpan is removed and covered with a disposable paper cover. If the patient is able to cleanse himself he should be permitted to do so. If too weak and ill, the nurse must clean the patient and leave him dry and comfortable. If necessary a clean sheet is inserted. The bedclothes are arranged properly and the patient is encouraged to wash his hands. The room should be aired. The contents of the bedpan are inspected by the nurse and reported upon, and saved, if necessary.

An enema may also be given with a tube and funnel.

Preparation of the Apparatus

A tray is required containing:

        Jug of tap water at 38°C (100°F)
        Funnel, tubing, connection and catheter (size 12) in a
            bowl

I

Linen or paper squares
Lubricant, e.g. Vaseline
Kidney dish
Paper bag for used swabs
Paper towel

together with a bedpan. The amount of the solution used depends on the age and physical condition of the patient. It ranges from 500 ml to 1000 ml.

Preparation of the Patient

This is the same as for giving a disposable enema.

The Technique

The apparatus is filled with fluid, to push out the air. The tube is nipped between the thumb and forefinger, to prevent it emptying. The catheter is lubricated and passed through the anus for about ten centimetres. Taking care not to allow air to enter, the funnel is filled. It is held about thirty centimetres above the level of the patient. The prescribed amount of fluid is used unless the patient complains of more than the usual slight and temporary discomfort. The tube is nipped and gently withdrawn. The catheter is detached and placed in a receiver. The patient is turned over and the bedpan placed under him.

The rest of the procedure is the same as for a disposable enema.

Dangers

If the solution used is too hot, there may be burning of the rectal mucosa—if too cold, shock might arise—and if air is introduced, pain will be complained of. Due to the distension of the rectum with fluid, the patient may feel faint, or collapse.

The contaminated hands of the nurse transfer disease organisms very easily. They should be washed thoroughly after handling the bedpan.

Regular use of enemas becomes habit forming, and after a time they are less effective.

Rectal Examination

For diagnostic purposes a rectal examination is made. A simple explanation is given to the patient. Privacy is ensured, and the patient placed in the left lateral position with the body flexed and the buttocks to the edge of the bed. The bedclothes are turned back but the patient is exposed as little as possible.

The doctor powders his hand if necessary and puts on the rubber glove, or finger stall with cape (disposable if possible). The index finger is lubricated. The patient is asked to relax and to breathe in and out through the mouth. The finger is inserted into the rectum. A bimanual examination may be made by placing the other hand on the abdomen.

At the conclusion of the examination the doctor withdraws his finger. The faeces on the glove, or finger stall, may be saved for laboratory testing. It is then wiped and discarded into a paper bag. If necessary the anus is wiped. The patient is made comfortable.

It must be remembered that these treatments may be embarrassing to the patient, therefore the nurse must guard against being too matter of fact, or affected by the patient's attitude.

FURTHER READING

Norton, Exton, Smith & McLaren, *An Investigation of Geriatric Nursing Problems in Hospital*. National Association for the Care of Old People.

Rudd, *The Nursing of the Elderly Sick*. Faber.

Taverner, *Physiology for Nurses*. E.U.P.

CHAPTER 14

THE NURSE'S RESPONSIBILITY
TOWARDS SPECIMENS

Every day on the wards the observant nurse sees very clearly that her patients' appearance and physical characteristics are altered by illness. This upset of the normal functioning of the body is also reflected in the excretions. The composition of the normal excretions is known. Specimens of the patient's excretions can be obtained and analysed or tested. Deviations from the normal are shown and in many cases these can be attributed to definite causes. Much very useful information is therefore obtained from examination of bodily excretions.

The nurse is not usually called upon to do the actual examination. This is the province of those who work in the various laboratories attached to the hospital. It is usually the nurse's responsibility to collect these specimens from the patient and see that they are delivered to the appropriate laboratory. In due course reports return to the ward and the nurse assures herself that these are filed with the patient's notes and seen by the doctor. In some cases it may be necessary to inform the doctor immediately of the result of an investigation. Often it can be left until his next visit to the patient. Only experience can tell the nurse which course of action to adopt.

Types of Containers

Because of the wide variety of tests which may be carried out on these specimens, different forms of containers are used for different excretions. Waxed paper or plastic boxes are commonly used for specimens of faeces, vomit or sputum. Blood and urine are usually collected in glass bottles, and specimens from the patient in the theatre are put into special dishes. Sometimes the containers are dry; sometimes they already contain a substance with which the specimen is immediately mixed. In every case it is most important that every container is labelled immediately a specimen is put into it. On the result of the investigation a great deal may depend, and it is obviously extremely important that reports should refer to the right patient. Labels must be clearly written and nurses must remember that there are often many patients in a hospital with similar names. Particulars must be carefully checked with the notes of the patient; especial care must be taken when dealing with common names such as Jones, Smith or Brown.

After the specimen has been collected and labelled it must go to the laboratory without undue delay. Some particular specimens must go immediately, otherwise they are useless. Others wait to be collected at a pre-arranged time.

COLLECTION OF SPECIFIC SPECIMENS

Urine

The appearance and characteristics of urine have already been noted. This is one excretion which the nurse examines on the ward using tablets or prepared papers.

Urine for testing must be collected in a clean, dry vessel. A man passes urine into a clean urinal and the urine is then poured into a tall vessel. A woman confined to bed uses a clean, dry bedpan and again the urine is transferred into a glass. A woman who is allowed to go to the lavatory can pass urine directly into a jug or jar. Most student nurses will have done this manoeuvre themselves during their medical examination on entry to the training school.

Swabbing of the vulva or penis beforehand allows a cleaner specimen of urine to be obtained. A further refinement is to ask the patient to start micturating, then collect the urine when it is flowing from the urethra. This midstream specimen is collected with greater ease from a man than a woman.

The abnormal constituents which may be found in urine are: albumin, blood, sugar, acetone, bile, pus. The requirements for testing urine are kept in a special cupboard which is usually in the sluice room or one of the ward annexes. All the equipment should be clean and the urine tested as soon as possible after voiding. The specific gravity is taken with a urinometer which floats in the urine. The reaction is tested with litmus paper. Red litmus paper turns blue in an alkaline fluid, blue litmus turns red in an acid. If neither paper shows a change the urine has a neutral reaction.

The tablets and papers used for testing must be fresh and the instructions for their use followed implicitly. Colour charts for comparison with the tests are provided and these give a straightforward assessment of the results of the tests.

24 *hour specimen*. Sometimes it is important to have not just a specimen of the urine tested but to examine the total 24 hour output. To do this a jar is obtained large enough to hold the urine, approximately 1½–2 litres. This is labelled with the patient's name and the date of collection. At a certain time, usually in the morning, the patient is asked to empty his bladder and this urine is thrown away. The test now starts with the patient having an empty bladder. All subsequent voidings are put in the jar which is kept covered. At the same hour on the following day the patient again empties his bladder, and this is the last addition to the jar.

Faeces

Normal faeces are brown in colour and solid or semi-solid in consistency. A large number of abnormal stools are seen in illness; this is not surprising when the length of the alimentary tract and the complexity of its secretions are considered.

The faeces vary in CONSISTENCY with the length of time the material is in the alimentary tract. If it hurries through, as in diarrhoea, then it is thin and watery. On the other hand, in constipation, when faecal material remains in the colon, the stool becomes hard and dry.

The COLOUR of the faeces is affected by a number of factors. Bile pigments normally confer on faeces their characteristic brown; if the pigments are diverted into other parts of the body, as in jaundice, the stool is very pale. If blood is present in the stomach, either escaping from an ulcer, or having been swallowed from a nose bleed, for example, that blood will be altered by the digestive juices. It will eventually appear in the faeces as a black tarry stool, known as melaena. On the other hand, bleeding from a lesion in the large colon or rectum will escape from the anus unaltered and will be seen as bright red blood in the stool.

In addition to consistency and colour the faeces may present a bizarre APPEARANCE because of abnormal additions. Foreign bodies such as coins, safety pins or even small toys may be seen. The stool may contain worms or part of a tape worm. The SMELL may also be altered or intensified. It is obvious, therefore, that although giving a patient a bedpan is not the most pleasant of duties, it is one which carries its own importance.

Collection of Specimens. Faecal specimens may either be transferred into a container or sent to the laboratory in the bedpan. Certain organisms, *e.g.*, Entamoeba Histolytica cannot survive long outside the warmth of the body, so stools which have to be examined for such organisms are accordingly taken straight to the laboratory in the bedpan whilst it is still warm, as it is much easier to identify the amoeba when it is still alive. The majority of faecal specimens are transferred from the bedpan to a waxed container. The nurse wears a disposable glove and uses a spatula. The container may either be sent to the laboratory as it is or put into a paper bag which facilitates handling.

Vomit

Urine and faeces, though they may contain abnormalities, are usual bodily excretions, vomit is not; but vomiting frequently occurs in illness, and observation of it may reveal much about the patient and his illness. There are innumerable causes of this symptom, ranging from the over-indulgence of a child in a favourite food to the intractable vomiting seen in some serious conditions such as intestinal obstruction. It is the doctor's responsibility to decide the cause of the sickness. It is the nurse's responsibility to report accurately upon it. The TIME of vomiting should be noted and the relationship between this and any other event. The patient might have been sick shortly after a meal, or he may have vomited on regaining consciousness after an operation. The AMOUNT should be noted, though this may not be an accurate measurement if the vomiting is unexpected and no receiver was at hand. The APPEARANCE should be noted. The vomit may consist of undigested food or it may be a greenish, watery fluid. If blood is in the stomach long enough to be altered by gastric juices it will be brown in colour and gritty in appearance, 'coffee grounds' being the traditional analogy.

The SOUND of vomiting can also vary. Some patients are sick with the maximum of retching and coughing, whilst others, usually more ill, allow the vomit to well up out of their mouths with hardly a sound. The actual vomiting may be preceded by nausea or it may occur suddenly and unexpectedly. The patient may complain of pain; sometimes this is relieved by vomiting, whilst sometimes being sick aggravates the pain.

Care of the Patient. In all cases of vomiting the nurse's first thought should be for the welfare of the patient. The curtains should be drawn round the bed, a bowl and cover provided and the patient's head supported. Any mess should be cleared away quickly and without fuss, and the patient's face sponged when the vomiting is over. A mouthwash is given and the dentures cleaned. After this the nurse should make a full and accurate report on the vomiting and save as much as she can for the ward sister, or sometimes the doctor, to see.

Sputum

In any gathering of English people coughing is so much part of the scene as to pass unnoticed. Indeed, many people would feel lost without their cough, but this should not hide the fact that a persistent cough is not normal. The respiratory system is a wonderfully engineered mechanism designed to get oxygen into the body and allow carbon dioxide to escape. The whole of the system is designed to cope with air, so if anything other than air is in the air passages the body will try to get rid of it—by coughing. If sputum is expelled, the cough is productive. If the irritating substance is very small in quantity or a vapour (*e.g.*, cigarette smoke) then the cough is hard and dry. Disease of the respiratory system is almost invariably accompanied by a cough, and in many instances characteristic sputum is produced. This varies very much in type and quantity. THIN SPUTUM is usually produced in quite large amounts and is fairly easily expelled. THICK TENACIOUS SPUTUM sometimes sticks to the bronchial tree and the patient is too weak to make the necessary great effort to dislodge it. If a lung abscess has formed or the patient has pockets of pus in his lungs, as in bronchiectasis, then the sputum will be infected. The smell is quite revolting both to the patient and the nurse. Blood may be coughed up—a most terrifying experience again to both parties. Whatever sputum is produced, collecting a specimen of it is an easy matter, as the patient simply coughs it into the appropriate container and this is then sent to the laboratory.

All these four secretions, urine, faeces, vomit and sputum are produced by the patient and the nurse has to collect a specimen. Nurses will find that in order to prove a diagnosis or assess a course of treatment, doctors use artificial means to obtain other specimens. Syringes and needles are used to withdraw blood or fluids from the various cavities of the body. Abscesses may be opened and specimens of pus obtained. Smears may be taken from mucous membranes and the cells in the smears examined. These cells may show changes due to early malignancy and thus cytology (the study of cells) is an important aid to the early diagnosis of cancer. In all these, the nurse is responsible for seeing that the correct container is at hand; that it is correctly labelled; and taken or sent to the right laboratory.

As has already been said, a great deal of information, much of it valuable and some of it vital, may be obtained from the examination of specimens. A great deal of time and effort is expended in hospital on this and there is a danger of regarding it as an end in itself. Nurses must not lose sight of the fact that every specimen belongs to a patient and the latter is the more important. What is a routine procedure of collection for the nurse may be either a frightening or an embarrassing ordeal for the patient, and nurses must not forget this. Explanation beforehand will do much to instil confidence and any questions the patient asks should either be answered or referred to sister. Nurses look after human beings who in the end are always more interesting than their specimen reports.

FURTHER READING

Lascelles and Donaldson, *Essential Diagnostic Tests*. Medical & Technical Publishing Co. Ltd.

Houghton and Gee, *Pocket Book of Ward Information*. Balliere, Tindall & Cassell.

Ross and Wilson, *Foundations of Anatomy and Physiology*. Livingstone.

CHAPTER 15

ASEPTIC TECHNIQUE OR PROTECTING THE PATIENT FROM INFECTION

Any disorder or unhealthy condition of the body is called a disease. One of the first ideas that came to our primitive ancestors was that disease was caused by evil spirits which entered into the person's body. Some primitive people still believe that disease can be cured by making a loud noise, or by causing pain —to scare it away.

It was not until the nineteenth century that Louis Pasteur, the great French scientist, showed that many diseases were caused by minute living organisms. Those which affect us are— bacteria (tiny single-celled plants), viruses, and protozoans (single-celled animals). They are found in air, water, soil, on animals and on humans, and some are enemies of man. Before Pasteur's work there were no known ways of protecting man from infection.

Joseph Lister, a Scottish surgeon, discovered antiseptics and was knighted by Queen Victoria for his brilliant contribution to medical science. His work was based on Pasteur's findings. Lister used a spray of carbolic acid and this killed the organisms. Unfortunately, the solution proved too drastic for the body substances, and living cells were damaged at first.

To-day, perfectly clean equipment, *i.e.*, sterile equipment, is used, and procedures are carried out with aseptic technique. This is widely practised wherever the sick are nursed.

Sterility

By *sterility* is meant the complete absence of all forms of life. A sterile article does not carry bacteria or micro-organisms— it is perfectly clean. In the operating theatre, for instance, sterile instruments and articles are prepared for the surgeon who uses them for all operations. The surgeon knows that however close they get to the patient, they cannot spread disease.

If a sterile article touches an unsterile object contamination will occur, that is, bacteria from the unsterile object will spread to the sterile one, which then ceases to be sterile.

To make articles sterile the use of heat in a specified time is by far the most reliable method in everyday use. Temperature and time can be accurately controlled. If heat cannot be applied, because the material to be sterilised would be damaged, it would be as well to use material that would stand up to heat and yet serve the same purpose.

Micro-organisms on the articles to be sterilized vary greatly in their resistance to different attempts at sterilization. Spore-forming bacteria require specific techniques. Bacteria which do not form spores can be got rid of in the simple ways of pasteurization and boiling.

Pasteurization is relied upon to kill all the micro-organisms found in milk, to make it safe for human consumption. When milk is heated to 71·5°C (161°F) and kept at this temperature for 30 seconds, bacteria are killed. Rapid cooling afterwards is an extra precaution.

Boiling. Articles to be sterilized by boiling should be placed in cold water and the temperature gradually raised. Wrapped or large articles may take time to reach the required temperature, *e.g.*, a needle with a stilette through the lumen, or instruments with threads or ratchets. Any vessel can be used, provided it is deep enough to allow the water to cover the articles, and can be heated sufficiently to boil the water. Deep saucepans can be used in homes. In hospitals 'sterilizers' may still be used. Lids should be fitted, the water must be kept boiling, and it must completely cover the articles all the time. THREE minutes is the time agreed by authorities for boiling, and these minutes should be timed with a watch or a clock, or an egg-timer provided for the purpose. If an egg-timer is placed on the lid, it will prevent the hasty person from upsetting the procedure. (It is clear from this that much heat and many hours have been wasted in the past when 'sterilizers' have been untouched for 20 minutes or longer!)

Use of steam under pressure. Destruction of spores cannot be achieved by the boiling of water in an open vessel, but it can be obtained by the use of steam under pressure. The highest temperature that water can reach when boiled in an open vessel is 100°C (212°F) but many housewives have found that if water is boiled in a completely closed vessel like a pressure cooker, so that the steam is under pressure, a very much higher temperature is reached.

In order to change water into steam a large amount of heat is needed, and some of this heat remains hidden (or becomes 'latent') within the steam. Articles inside a pressure chamber— a housewife's pressure cooker, or a hospital's autoclave—become saturated with the steam, and as it condenses, the heat, which has been stored up, is given out again. Latent heat liberated in this way gives the sterilizing efficiency to the steam.

Time and temperature are still essential factors in moist heat sterilization, especially with steam under pressure. Articles exposed to 100°C (212°F) are freed of all vegetative bacteria and viruses within a few seconds, but spores will not be destroyed.

To destroy spores it is necessary to employ 121°C (250°F) for 20 minutes.

It is necessary for air to be removed from the pressure chamber, and the articles within it, and for live steam to take its place. As air is almost twice as heavy as steam it can be pushed out through an opened valve in the bottom part of an autoclave, or it can be pumped out. With the doors and valves closed, both the pressure and the temperature of the steam, within the chamber, will gradually rise. Depending upon the 'load' within the chamber, when the pressure reaches:

10 lb per square inch the temperature should be 116°C (240°F)

15 lb per square inch the temperature should be 121°C (250°F)

When the required pressure has been reached no more steam is allowed in. This temperature and pressure is maintained for 20 minutes. Generally a safety valve will blow if the pressure rises above 15 lb per square inch. A vacuum is now produced by releasing the steam from the chamber. It is not possible to open the doors because of the vacuum inside, so twice-filtered air is allowed in to restore the interior to atmospheric pressure and to cool and dry the load. After this the doors can be opened and sterilized articles removed. If the contents of the autoclave are not completely dry at the end of the process, they should not be used. The load, in these circumstances, must be regarded as unsafe.

A short simple summary of the working of an autoclave is:
1. Check containers
2. Load shelves
3. Close autoclave
4. Create vacuum

5. Raise pressure to required level
6. Maintain pressure at given level, for stated time
7. Extract steam
8. Dry contents
9. Check chart
10. Open autoclave (wearing mask and protective gloves)
11. Close, and remove containers.

Cotton fabrics, nylon, rubber, instruments, watery solutions and water can be sterilized in this way. The steam passes from above downwards, therefore the packing of containers should allow for vertical spaces in between articles. The position of containers in the pressure chamber is also an important factor in allowing adequate sterilization.

Laboratory technicians can prove the efficiency of autoclaves by the use of specially prepared tubes, or papers, containing bacterial spores. Tests will show that the most resistant spores are killed at a temperature of 121°C (250°F) at a pressure of 15 lb per square inch, in 20 minutes.

High vacuum high pressure autoclaves are now in use in many hospitals. The chamber is much smaller than in the conventional autoclave, and by using a pump a vacuum of 29 inches is rapidly produced. Steam is allowed in at 32 lb per square inch, giving a temperature of 134°C (273°F) for $3\frac{1}{2}$ minutes, the procedure is controlled by pressing buttons.

Dry heat. Substances and articles that cannot be penetrated by steam, *e.g.*, powders and oils, require dry heat sterilization. Syringes and glassware and instruments also can be treated in a HOT AIR OVEN. A heat of 160°C (322°F) is reached before the timing is started, when one hour is allowed. There must be free circulation of hot air between the articles in the hot air oven.

Infra-red radiation of syringes, in a syringe service, is a satisfactory alternative to the hot air oven.

Gamma Radiation. Many pre-packed articles are sterilized by gamma radiation at Atomic Energy Centres, and are in general use in hospitals.

Chemicals. If chemicals are to be used for sterilization they must be able to act:
(a) on any type of micro-organism
(b) within a known time, *i.e.*, from a few seconds to 30 minutes,

(c) in a known concentration

(d) in the presence of blood, pus, faeces, etc. (commonly called 'organic matter')

(e) without injuring the skin, damaging metals, or causing irritating vapours.

Many chemicals are prepared commercially and much is claimed for them, but as yet no one chemical is available that will fulfil all the requirements stated above.

There are many groups of chemicals and further study is essential if details are to be known.

The gas—formaldehyde may be used for disinfection of rooms and furniture, and is more effective if used at a high temperature.

Keeping Articles Sterile—Storage and Handling

It has been seen that specific methods are used to make sure that articles and substances are made free of all living matter. Once this state of sterility has been reached the many different containers must be unsealed only when about to be used.

Many hospitals have Central Sterile Supplies Departments, the staff of which are responsible for issuing containers and packets to wards and departments. Containers and packets are generally sealed with test-tape which goes brown on being heated. Equipment for two or three days' supply is generally kept on the ward, special equipment being obtained when it is needed.

A nurse has to learn how to open packs, and remove foil caps, carefully, to prevent contamination. Methods vary in hospitals, but the principles are the same. The contents of the containers and packets are either picked up with sterile forceps, or carefully emptied into a sterile gallipot or dish. Practice under supervision will provide the necessary dexterity.

Contamination will be caused if the articles inside the containers come into contact with anything that is not sterile, especially air, water, or the hands of the nurse or doctor. Torn or wet packets must never be used.

Techniques can now be performed without any risk of spreading disease, provided that nurses and doctors do not fail in their own personal responsibilities.

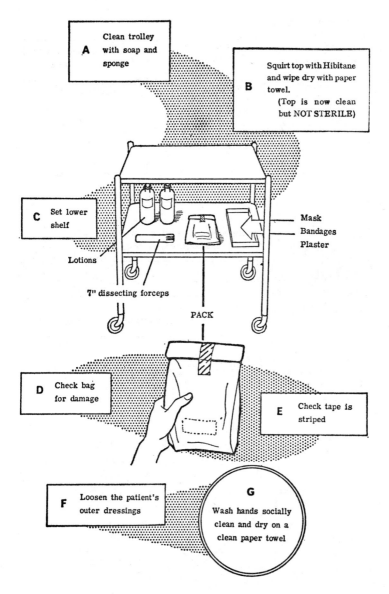

A   Clean trolley with soap and sponge

B   Squirt top with Hibitane and wipe dry with paper towel.
(Top is now clean but NOT STERILE)

C   Set lower shelf

Mask
Bandages
Plaster

Lotions

7" dissecting forceps

PACK

D   Check bag for damage

E   Check tape is striped

F   Loosen the patient's outer dressings

G   Wash hands socially clean and dry on a clean paper towel

FIG. 50 One example of requirements for a dressing trolley, using C.S.S.D. equipment

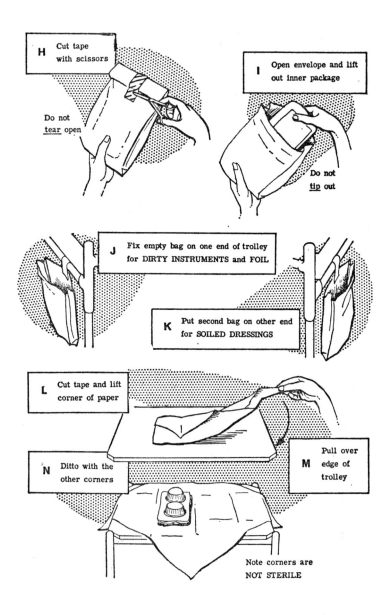

H Cut tape with scissors

Do not <u>tear</u> open

I Open envelope and lift out inner package

Do not <u>tip</u> out

J Fix empty bag on one end of trolley for DIRTY INSTRUMENTS and FOIL

K Put second bag on other end for SOILED DRESSINGS

L Cut tape and lift corner of paper

N Ditto with the other corners

M Pull over edge of trolley

Note corners are NOT STERILE

FIG. 51 Opening the pack

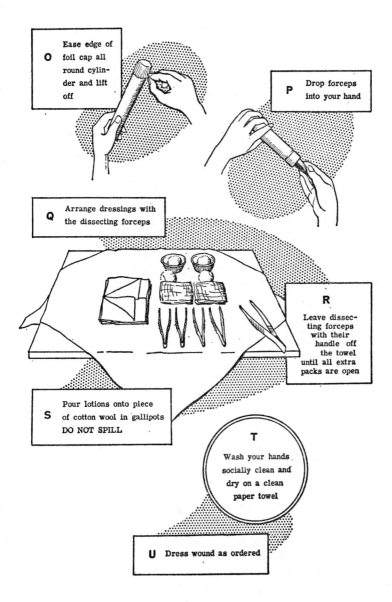

O Ease edge of foil cap all round cylinder and lift off

P Drop forceps into your hand

Q Arrange dressings with the dissecting forceps

R Leave dissecting forceps with their handle off the towel until all extra packs are open

S Pour lotions onto piece of cotton wool in gallipots DO NOT SPILL

T Wash your hands socially clean and dry on a clean paper towel

U Dress wound as ordered

FIG. 52 Setting the trolley

K

CLEARING UP

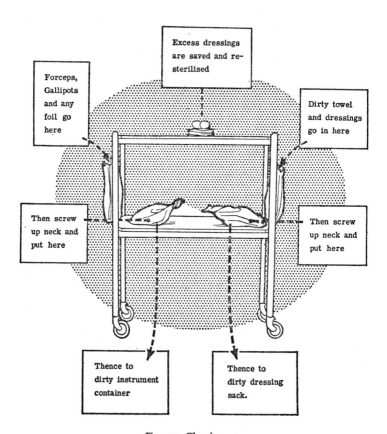

Fig. 53 Clearing up

FURTHER READING

Hare, *Bacteriology and Immunity for Nurses*. Longmans.
Ludovici, *The World of the Infinitely Small*. Phoenix. House.
Williams, Blowers, Garrod and Shooter, *Hospital Infection, Causes and Prevention*. Lloyd Luke.
Winner, H. I., *Microbiology in Modern Nursing*. E.U.P.

CHAPTER 16

CROSS INFECTION AND THE NURSE

When Florence Nightingale said 'The hospital should do the patient no harm' she was probably not thinking of cross infection, but in a modern hospital some of the greatest harm done to patients is to pass infection to them whilst they are being treated. This passage of infection in air, dust, on a common object or by direct contact from one person in the ward to another is known as cross infection, and its consequences can be very serious indeed.

A patient admitted for a minor operation may have infection passed to him from another patient which will prolong his stay in hospital, dislocate all his arrangements (he may have arranged for a substitute to do his job), prevent him from earning again for a longer period than he expected and block the bed so that other patients' admission may be delayed. Hospital care is very expensive and each extra day a patient spends in hospital adds to the nation's hospital bill. Infection, with resultant delay in healing, may also cause scarring of a wound that should have healed cleanly and in cases of plastic surgery this may ruin the result of the operation.

Apart from the organisms causing known infectious diseases, the bacteria which are potentially the most dangerous are certain of the staphylococci, the bacillus coli and others such as the pseudomonas pyocyaneus. Staphylococci are organisms which are commonly found on the skin, they cause boils and styes and other pus-producing lesions. They are not all harmful but some of them have learnt to adapt themselves to resist the action of antibiotics and are therefore very dangerous. Bacillus coli are harmless in the colon, but may cause chronic infection in the urinary tract and elsewhere. The word 'pathogenic' is used to describe harmful bacteria.

Method of Spread

An infected person, according to the type of infecting organism can spread infection from his nose and mouth (droplet infection), in his faeces and urine (in this case often indirectly on his hands), or from a wound or lesion on his skin. Infection can enter the body through the nose and mouth (inhalation), through the mouth (ingestion) and through the skin if it is broken (inoculation). The important factors for the nurse to be aware of are how infection spreads from one person to the other.

Droplet infection may spread directly through the air—'coughs and sneezes spread diseases'—but more usually the bacteria cling to particles of dust, infecting the area where the dust lies and spreading into the air again when the dust is disturbed. Any article used or handled by the patient must be regarded as potentially infected, thus all linen, crockery, cutlery, toilet articles, toys, etc. could carry infection to another person

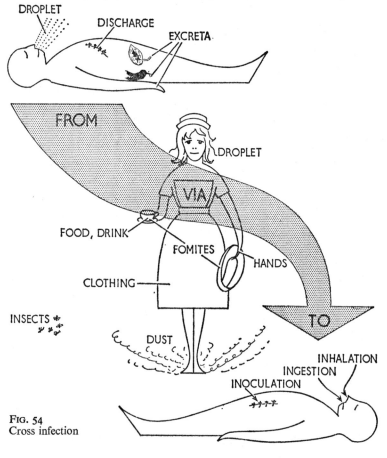

FIG. 54
Cross infection

unless disinfected. These potentially infected objects are sometimes referred to as fomites. Infection can be carried by insects
or by infected food and drink, but this is unlikely in a hospital
ward. A more likely way for infection to spread from one patient
to another is for it to be carried directly by the nurse. Nurses
can carry infection because of faulty technique, but they may also
carry dangerous bacteria in their noses or throats without
being aware of it. A person who carries infection, but is not
affected by it himself, is called a 'carrier'.

The Responsibility of the Nurse

The nurse has three main responsibilities in preventing the
spread of infection. She must see that the general level of bacteria
in the ward is kept as low as possible, whether harmless or
harmful. She must make sure that she has intelligent understanding of the ways in which specific infections are spread, so
that she herself is never responsible for introducing or carrying
infection in the ward.

*On the integrity of the individual nurse does the safety of the
patient depend.* She is the one who must realize that to go on
duty with a boil or stye or even a heavy cold, is as dangerous to
her patients as the pus from another patient's wound. She must
be responsible, without continual reminders, for the cleanliness
of her uniform, the care of her finger nails, the tidy dressing of
her hair. Any nurse who does not believe that bacteria may be
carried on soiled aprons, under long finger nails and on flopping
hair, should take the opportunity to grow some on an agar plate
and see. She is the only person who knows whether or not her
infectious precautions have been properly carried out. There is
no place for those whose motto is 'thou shalt not be found out'.
Every nurse, however junior, has an equal responsibility where
these techniques are concerned. One careless nurse can break
the invisible barrier set up by ten conscientious ones.

General Precaution Against Infection

Bacteria like warm, moist, dark places, so a light, well-ventilated
ward will help to reduce their numbers. All surfaces which collect
dust, such as shelves and working tops, should be made of material which is easily washed. Dust should be kept to a minimum
by mopping and dusting with special mops and cloths which,

in their turn, should be washed regularly. Linen articles, which are potential spreaders of infection, should be replaced by paper; for example, hand towels and bedpan covers. All other ward linen, such as bed curtains and bedding, should be made of material which it is possible to boil. Cotton blankets, for example, are more suitable than woollen ones. Although they carry about equal numbers of bacteria, it is impossible to boil a woollen blanket without reducing its usefulness as a blanket. Articles such as dish clothes and tea towels should be eliminated altogether, either by the use of washing-up machines, or by using water so hot that crockery and cutlery dry themselves. Pillows and mattresses should have washable covers.

Special Precautions Against Infection

If a patient does develop an infection whilst in a general ward, the ideal is to move him to an isolation unit, or failing this, to a side ward. However, this is not always possible, and many infectious patients have to be nursed in the general ward, when a technique known as 'barrier nursing' is used. The general principles of 'barrier nursing' technique are simple. The nurses, in effect, create an invisible barrier round the patient's bed and prevent infection reaching either themselves or any of the other patients. There is no particular magical ritual about barrier nursing, any nurse, however junior, can carry it out, provided she knows in each case how the infection is spread from each patient she nurses. For example, if the infection is spread by droplets, it will be particularly important to wear a mask; if it is spread in the faeces, use of a mask will be unnecessary, but handwashing will be all-important.

All barrier techniques have a certain amount in common and are then adapted for the individual patient and the particular way in which his infection is spread.

Patient Nursed in the Ward

The bed should be in a corner, near the sluice if possible. A screen should be placed at the foot of the bed to serve as a reminder to other patients and staff. Outside the screen should hang the gowns which nurses and doctors must wear when attending to the patient. These gowns are to protect the clothing of the wearer, and should be donned with great care, keeping the 'clean' inside of the gown next to the wearer, and tying the tapes firmly so that the clothing is properly covered. When attention has been given to the patient, the nurse's hands are 'dirty' and she must therefore wash them before untying the 'clean' tapes of her gown. She next slides out of the gown, hanging it on its hanger with the 'dirty' side inmost, and then washes her hands

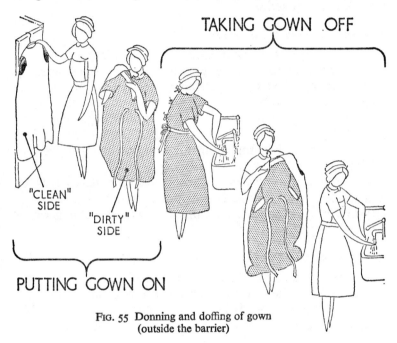

TAKING GOWN OFF

"CLEAN" SIDE

"DIRTY" SIDE

PUTTING GOWN ON

Fig. 55 Donning and doffing of gown
(outside the barrier)

again. This is easy to remember if the nurse knows that the 'clean' inside of the gown always touches her uniform and is exposed to the ward side of the barrier, and the 'dirty' outside of her gown is only exposed to the patient.

If masks or gloves are required they are provided outside the barrier. Disposable masks are the easiest to use, but nurses should resist the temptation to screw them up in their hands after removal. They should be lifted off by the ear pieces and placed in a paper bag ready for burning later. If they are of the disposable type, gloves are thrown away after use. If not, they are washed on the hands and used again; they are for the protection of the nurse, and need not be sterile.

Each infectious patient should keep his own personal belongings such as thermometer, washing things, medicine glass, etc., inside the barrier. Articles which are normally kept in the kitchen (crockery or cutlery), or in the sluice (bedpans and urinals) should either be kept in a special 'barrier' sluice and 'barrier' kitchen, or sterilized immediately after use and stored in the ward kitchen or sluice.

Patient Nursed in a Side Ward

It is often simpler to nurse a patient in a side ward, as it is easier to keep his personal belongings near him, and trays, washing bowls, etc. may be stored more conveniently than in the ward. The gowns can also be kept inside the room, and the nurse must remember that in this case their 'dirty' side is kept outermost. Most side wards have a wash basin, but if not, a bowl of water must be provided in the room for hand-washing before and after removing the gown.

An outline of the ways in which infected material may be dealt with is given below. Nurses must know how infection is spread from their patient, and employ only those methods which are necessary in each case.

Disposal of Infected Linen

A suitable container is brought to the bedside, an example is a plastic bin on wheels with a plastic bag as a 'liner'. Infected linen is dropped into this inner bag, without handling the bin at all, it is then wheeled back to the sluice. There the inner 'liner' is removed and later collected. The bag should be clearly labelled 'infectious' before it leaves the ward. On reaching the laundry it is treated in some way (either soaked in disinfectant or fumigated) before being laundered. In an emergency linen is perfectly safe if treated in a disinfectant such as formalin solution 1:250 for 30 minutes before being sent to the laundry, but this is not ideal, as the handling of infectious material should be reduced to a minimum.

Disposal of Infected Faeces

In a country such as Great Britain where there is an adequate main drainage system, it is not necessary to disinfect faeces before flushing them down the sluice. The bedpan, however, still remains a potential source of infection and should be rinsed and then sterilized, either by soaking in disinfectant, or by boiling. After dealing with a bedpan the nurse should wash her hands with great care. In places where the drainage system is not adequate, faeces may be soaked in disinfectant such as formalin solution 1:250 for one hour before flushing them away; the bedpan is then dealt with separately.

Disposal of Infected Crockery and Cutlery

All food scraps from the infectious plate should be scraped into a paper bag and burnt. In some cases it may be possible for the patient's crockery to be washed in a special sink and kept for his use alone, if not, it should be sterilized and kept in the ward kitchen with the general stock. An efficient dish-washer will sterilize all crockery and cutlery. Paper plates and cups, together with plastic cutlery may be used as these are completely disposable.

Disposal of Infected Sputum

Sputum should be collected in a paper carton and burnt. An alternative is to autoclave a metal sputum mug and its contents before cleansing it.

Other Articles

Other articles used at the bedside are many and include thermometers, tooth mugs, washing bowls, tooth brushes, stethoscopes, pulsometers, books, toys, etc. These must all be disinfected or destroyed. Those articles which cannot be boiled must be soaked in disinfectant. Those which cannot be soaked must be fumigated by exposing them to disinfectant gas. Mattresses and pillows may be damaged by fumigation so are often used with waterproof covers which can be washed. If not, they *must* be fumigated, but nurses should remember to air them well afterwards.

When the period of infection is over all articles used by the patient, together with his bed and bedding (not forgetting the bed curtains) must be sterilized appropriately. The patient himself, after bathing and washing his hair, is placed in a clean bed with clean linen.

Loopholes

There are many points at which barrier technique may break down unless the nurse is vigilant. The patient himself may not understand that he is infectious, and pass his daily paper to his neighbour in the usual friendly way. Other patients and visitors may not realize the significance of the screen and walk in and sit down for a chat. This is not to say the patient must be forbidden visitors, his isolation makes him very lonely and depressed, but they must wear proper protective clothing, and wash their hands when leaving the barrier in the usual way. Doctors and medical students create another problem; donning a barrier gown in the correct manner does not seem to be part of the medical student's curriculum, and many senior men seem to possess magic self-sterilizing stethoscopes. Ward maids and cleaners have to be taught the special methods of cleansing infected rooms. Indeed, the dusting and sweeping during the infectious period may even be assigned to the nurse. But the last loophole is the nurse herself. She must remember that ordinary soap and water and high general standards of cleanliness, together with a little common sense, are more important than half-remembered rituals inaccurately carried out because their purpose has been forgotten. Nurses often think that because an object is rendered sterile by a certain disinfectant in half an hour, it is somehow MORE sterile if left in for twelve hours. She will wipe a salt cellar with elaborate care, but may thoughtlessly enter the cubicle with long dirty nails or flopping hair which may readily infect the next patient she cares for, or the next wound she dresses. It must never be forgotten that the nurse has the greatest chance to spread infection in the ward, and it is on the integrity of each individual nurse that the safety of the patient depends.

FURTHER READING

Hare, *Bacteriology and Immunity for Nurses*. Longmans.
Williams, Blowers, Garrod and Shooter, *Hospital Infection, Causes and Prevention*. Lloyd Luke.
Winner, H. I., *Microbiology in Modern Nursing*. E.U.P.

CHAPTER 17

THE CHILD IN HOSPITAL

This chapter is not intended for nurses who wish to specialise in paediatric nursing, but as an introduction to the subject for those who have to work in a children's ward during their general training. Nurses who have had no previous contact with young children may find the general remarks more helpful than those who are used to dealing with younger brothers and sisters, but all will find there are certain differences in nursing technique which are important to learn about.

Children in Hospital

A hospital is not a natural environment for children, and there is always a risk of emotional side effects from their stay. Children under five are particularly vulnerable, those under three being at the greatest risk. Because of this, every effort is made to keep young children out of hospital altogether or at least reduce their stay to a minimum. Many hospitals admit children as day cases for simple surgery or, if their stay has to be prolonged, the mother is admitted with the child. If the lack of suitable child/mother accommodation or the claims of other children at home make this impossible, free visiting is the only alternative. A well run children's ward has parents and visitors about at all times.

The Nurse and the Parents

One of the first lessons that nurses have to learn is that no amount of fondness for children, even if coupled with professional skill, will ever make a nurse as important or necessary to a child as his mother. Nurses make very good mother substitutes, but a substitute is not quite the same as the real thing! A nurse who has never had a child cannot fully appreciate the depth of a mother's anxiety or enter into any guilt feelings about the cause of the child's illness, but a good nurse knows that these feelings exist and takes them into account when planning her nursing care. All nursing skills connected with caring for a child must therefore include caring for his mother with tact and gentleness. The nurse and the mother must work closely together, but it is up to the nurse to be aware of those feelings of jealousy and frustration which may arise between herself and the mother, and look at the situation objectively. Two factors which increase the mother's anxiety and tension are ignorance and frustration at being unable to help her child. If she is allowed to express her fears freely, her questions are answered and her advice is heeded (she is after all the expert in the care of her child) she will find it easier to relax and help the nursing staff.

Although the main task of supporting and advising parents falls to sister and the doctor, the junior nurse is the one who finds herself most often the person who does things for the child in front of his mother. As her own techniques may not be very expert, she may feel considerable anxiety if the mother comments unfavourably or questions what she is doing. 'The other nurse never does that' may make her very flustered, and the more flustered she becomes the more she may find herself trying to discount what the mother is saying and asserting that she (the nurse) is in the right. If there is any doubt it is always better to check with someone more senior, but the important thing is that the child does not suffer because of tensions between nurse and mother.

Information

Both parents and child will need explanations of what is to happen to the child. Sister and the doctor will deal with more serious matters, but nurses must always be ready to give a simple explanation of what they are about to do for the child and why. Explanations are usually given to the mother first, out of earshot of the child, then either nurse or mother makes the final explanation. There are two points to remember, children should always be told the truth, (though not necessarily in great detail) and the language used should be very simple.

Children are apt to take explanations quite literally, interpreting them in the light of their own limited experience. This is especially true of half heard scraps of information, often not intended for their ears. The child who saw some 'bad' meat crawling with maggots and subsequently heard that he had a 'bad heart' assumed that his heart was crawling with maggots and became very distressed.

As no adult can guess what is going on in a child's mind, nurses must become skilled in helping children to express their thoughts, keeping an 'inner ear' open for the meaning of the seemingly casual remarks children make. 'Will I wake up after the operation' should never be dismissed with 'yes of course' but countered with 'Why do you ask?' It may then be discovered that the child has learnt he will be 'put to sleep' and imagines he will meet the same fate as the family cat. It is necessary to try to find the cause of a child's anxiety before reassuring him.

It is important that when treatments are carried out and drugs given, anything which is unpleasant or painful should not be glossed over. If an injection has to be given the reason should always be explained, 'This is to take the pain away', the fact that it is painful mentioned, 'You must be very brave because it is going to be sore', and the injection given swiftly. The child may then be comforted.

PROMISES SHOULD NEVER BE GIVEN UNLESS THEY CAN BE KEPT. When uncertain the nurse should say 'I will try but I can't promise' remembering that very young children cannot even understand promises unless they are fulfilled immediately. 'Mummy will come after tea' can be understood by a five year old but a three year old has no concept of time and this is no comfort to him. It is necessary to be careful about non verbal promises; to a toddler, having a bib tied round his neck means lunch and if it doesn't come straight away he will complain.

Working with Children

Normal children grow and develop by exploring and questioning their environment. They are constantly stimulated by interested adults at home and at school as well as by the happenings of every day life. When the child enters hospital every effort must be made for his normal development to continue unchecked, and as far as possible the hospital should be geared to the needs of the child and not the other way round. Nurses do not always have time to play with children as much as the children need being played with, so there is a special staff of play ladies and school teachers who all help to keep the child amused and occupied.

Most children are brave and co-operative about being in hospital, especially if they sense that parents and nurses are working together. Nurses should try and provide a certain framework of ward routine in a background of loving approval. There is however a great temptation to set artificial standards, and relate good and bad behaviour entirely to the degree of trouble caused to the ward staff. Thus a very unhappy withdrawn toddler may be dismissed as 'good' and ignored, whereas another may be told he is 'bad' for singing joyfully during the consultant's round. It is also important that nurses do not fall into the common error of supposing that because children 'play up' when their parents arrive it means that nurses are better at managing them. Children always behave better with strangers and control themselves more tightly in a strange environment, it is only with those they really love that they feel safe enough to express their feelings.

All children need to know they are loved. With older children the nurse must be sensitive to their feelings, some like open expressions of affection, others do not; but with young children and babies kissing and cuddling are as necessary to their recovery as medicine. Indeed some units allow nurses to wear mufti so they can work unhampered by spikey badges and starched aprons.

There is one patient however, who may be anything but cooperative, as his mother will tell the nurse, and that is the two year old. He has just made the intoxicating discovery that he is leading an independent existence. In order to assert this independence his answer to any sort of suggestion may well be a firm unequivocal 'NO'. The only way to handle him is by guile. Mothers and nurses usually insist on certain points of behaviour, e.g. he should never go into the lift alone, but if they are clever they do not make an issue out of non essentials. Most two year olds can be made to do what is wanted by a judicious mixture of removal of temptation and distraction. For example an ophthalmoscope should not be left where he can reach it, but if he does get hold of one, it must be retrieved by offering a toy in fair exchange. The nurse must try to see the world from his point of view. If he is found dipping his toothbrush in the lavatory before cleaning his teeth, he may be congratulated on his efforts but the nurse explains that the wash basin is better and places a chair so that he can reach it. If the nurse appears upset about this use of the lavatory he will keep on trying to find out why she is cross. Fortunately children prefer approval to disapproval and like to 'do what everyone else does' but obvious displeasure should be reserved for things that are really dangerous. The two year old will always continue to test adults, he is anxious to know whether they love him enough to make it safe for him to hate them.

Children and Food

Tempting a sick child to eat is one of the arts of paediatric nursing. Children are very conservative in their eating habits, and like familiar food served in a familiar way. A three year old was once made to start eating by an astute ward maid who tipped his chips into newspaper! Sometimes a child will eat something if it has been cooked by his mother, either at home and brought in, or in the ward kitchen. This is especially true if the child is used to special dishes like curry. Often a child may accept food from a ward maid or another child's parent when he will not take it from a nurse.

Nursing Procedures

When carrying out procedures in the children's ward, apart from the fact that the equipment is scaled down to child size there are many hazards and adaptations of technique. A few of these are set out below.

Admission of a Patient

A young child cannot be prepared for admission to hospital, unless his mother is able to stay with him, as he will immediately assume that she has left him for ever and mourn his loss. An older child can be well prepared by the use of books and stories about hospital. There is an excellent 'Ladybird' book available and some hospitals have their own comics or booklets which the child and his parents can read together before admission.

The information collected at the time of admission is normally obtained from the parents. With one or two additions, it is the same as for an adult. The nurse should find out:—Has the child any special likes or dislikes, has he any allergies to food or drugs? Has he been in contact with infectious disease recently? Which infections has he had? Is he up to date with his immunization programme?

In a younger child still speaking his own brand of English it is useful to know how he asks for a pottie. There is a wide range of nursery words for defaecation and micturition and nurses must not assume that the child will use the ones with which she is familiar.

Most toddlers have a special love object from which they refuse to be parted in time of trouble, particularly at night. This is usually some battered old toy or filthy rag (its owner will not usually part with it for long enough for it to be washed). The powerful influence of this 'familiar' is essential in the alarming world of hospital and the wise nurse makes sure it remains with its owner at all times. It is also useful to learn its name which tends to be idiosyncratic!

It is important to know whether or not a child has been christened and how the parents feel about this. Some may be comforted to know that the hospital chaplain will christen their baby if they wish, others hold different views which must be respected.

Drugs

Nurses who feel quite confident about giving drugs in an adult ward may find the doses in the children's ward so unfamiliar that they feel a certain lack of confidence at first. It is helpful if all staff, even state registered nurses, can be supervised by a paediatric nurse when they first give drugs in a children's ward until they become used to this difference. If a mistake were to be made its consequences could be more serious in a child. IF THERE IS ANY DOUBT CONSULT SISTER OR STAFF NURSE.

All children will have been labelled on admission and their bands must be checked before administration of a drug. When children are being nursed in cubicles there should be a planned agreed routine for giving drugs so that there is no confusion between the nurse in the cubicle and the nurses doing the drug round.

Two nurses should of course administer the drugs together and there will then be two people to hold the child when he is having an injection. The exception to this rule is the diabetic child who gives himself his own injections from an early age, and would scorn assistance.

Intravenous Fluids

Intravenous fluids, though life saving, may be very hazardous indeed for children. The total blood volume of a new born infant is the equivalent of half a pint of beer (300 mls), so it must be realised that the dangers of overloading the circulation are very great. If an infant is ordered a transfusion of 30 mls he must get 30 mls and no more. For this reason 'infant giving sets' are available with special counting chambers so that the rate of flow and the amount transfused can be carefully controlled. In infants the needle is usually in a vein in the scalp, in older children it is in a limb vein, but carefully guarded to prevent it being dislodged.

Infection

Children, especially babies, have less resistance to infection than adults. Infants and very sick children are nursed with barrier precautions to protect them from infection. Nurses must remember that though they may plan to carry out as many procedures as possible whilst in a cubicle, the hands must always be washed after changing, and before feeding, a baby.

Observations

All observations are made for a purpose, but those on the childrens ward are of vital importance. Firstly because children cannot always tell about their symptoms, and secondly because their condition can change very rapidly from apparent health to serious illness in a few hours. The doctor relies on the nurse and the mother to report any changes immediately.

Dangers

As every mother knows, children are at risk from dangers which no longer threaten adults. Parents gradually prepare the child to accept risks, relaxing their precautions as the child

L

learns such skills as using a knife or coming down stairs on his own. Hospitals who care for other people's children have to take more extreme precautions than individual parents. The most obvious dangers are of fire, falling, injestion of poisons and drowning. A few 'do's and don'ts' are listed below.

Do replace cot sides immediately.

Do tie restrainers (if used) to the frame of the cot not the sliding side piece.

Do stay with a child in the bathroom at all times.

Do be sure the child never leaves the ward alone.

Do make the ward toddler proof, (all cupboards above child height etc.).

Do make sure that no drugs or lotions used in treatments are ever left accessible to a child.

Do keep thermometer pots out of reach.

Do keep the kitchen and treatment room out of bounds.

This may seem rather a formidable list but nurses should not let it deter them from enjoyment of the childrens ward. The children very soon put everyone at ease. Once the nurse has got used to working with parents and children as a unit she will find it a very satisfying relationship and one day when she has children of her own she will accompany them to hospital with cheerful confidence.

FURTHER READING

Bowley, *The Psychological Care of the Child in Hospital.* Livingstone.

Duncombe and Weller, *Aids to Paediatric Nursing.* Balliere, Tindall & Cassell.

Rayner, *Mother and Midwives.* Allen & Unwin.

Robertson, *Children in Hospital.* Gollancz.

CHAPTER 18

PRE- AND POST-OPERATIVE CARE

A large number of people come into hospital because they are to have operations. These range from quite minor procedures to extensive complicated surgery, and the patient may be any age from 0 to 100. He may be admitted as an emergency requiring immediate operation; he may come to have a previously recommended operation or he may have an operation in the course of a long period of hospital treatment. In every case, however, there are two fundamental facts which nurses must not forget:

Every patient has a certain amount of fear about his operation.
Every operation, however small, carries a certain element of risk.

Mental Preparation

To deal with the first, nurses must remember that many patients will not disclose their fears and will not mention them unless prompted to do so. The amount of apprehension is not related to the severity of the operation, in fact the reverse is often the case. Temperament and character have much to do with the patient's approach to surgery, and reassurance is vital. This is best given by the ward atmosphere; a well-run and orderly ward with competent and friendly nurses is far more reassuring than frequent admonitions of 'You will be alright'. Other patients in the ward can be of tremendous help or incalculable harm. Nurses should assess their patients and encourage the former whilst tactfully protecting the new admission from the latter. The nature and extent of the operation should be explained to the patient, and this is the responsibility of the medical staff; the patient frequently asks questions, and these should be dealt with by the ward sister. It is both legally and morally wrong to operate on a patient or give him an anaesthetic until he has given his consent. This is obtained in writing and nurses must see that this has been done. In the case of a patient who is a minor the parents' consent must be obtained. Many patients derive strength and comfort from their religion and all of them should be given the opportunity to see their chaplain before the operation.

Physical Preparation

Every operation carries an element of risk, but that risk can be reduced to a minimum by careful pre-operative care.

Investigation

Careful examination of the patient is necessary to exclude any other illness or disability. This is carried out by the doctor but the nurse assists by examining the urine; by taking and recording the temperature, pulse and respiration; and by reporting any sign she notices or any symptom of which the patient complains.

Cleanliness

Absolute cleanliness reduces the risk of infection, thus hair should be shaved from the area of operation. This is done by nurses on female patients but pubic shaves on male patients are carried out by a male nurse or barber. The patient should then have a bath and extra care should be given to the umbilicus and the folds and clefts of the body. Sometimes the area of operation receives an extra cleansing with spirit followed by the application of an antiseptic; whether this is done or not depends on the wishes of the particular surgeon. If time and circumstances allow, the patient is more comfortable if the hair can be washed before operation. This is especially appreciated if the operation is in such a site that shampooing afterwards is difficult. The mouth should be clean; before extensive planned surgery a visit to the dentist is recommended.

Physiotherapy

Following operations and anaesthetics many patients develop coughs and respiratory infections. To prevent these, the physiotherapist should teach the patient breathing exercises, as well as leg and general exercises, before the operation. Smoking should be discouraged.

Management of Stomach and Bowel

One of the bigger risks is that the patient may inhale vomit during the administration of the anaesthetic. The stomach must be empty before the anaesthetic is given. In an emergency it may be necessary to pass a tube into the stomach and aspirate its contents. Otherwise it is sufficient to ensure that the patient has had no food or fluids for a period of four hours before he goes to the theatre. All patients must be told not to eat or drink during this time. Nurses should remember that many people do not think of sweets as food and these should be removed from the locker if nurses feel that the patient may take them.

For most operations it is desirable that the patient should not be constipated. If necessary this is accomplished by giving the patient a laxative or suppositories, but in no case should the nurse give these without instructions. Laxatives given to patients with some abdominal conditions may have disastrous consequences. Operations on the large bowel or rectum require careful preparation which will be specifically ordered.

Immediate Preparation

About an hour before the scheduled time of operation the final preparations are made. The patient empties his bladder; before some operations a catheter may be passed and left in position. A special gown is put on; this opens down the back and allows easy access to the operation site. Hair clips are removed and the hair is covered with a paper cap and the patient takes out any dentures. Any other artificial aid, such as contact lenses or a limb, would be removed. Jewellery is taken off and given to sister for safe keeping, though if married women like to wear their wedding rings they are allowed to as long as they are covered with strapping. Nail varnish and lipstick should be removed as colour of nails and lips is a valuable indication of the patient's condition.

The patients' label, which was fastened round his wrist when he was admitted, is checked. If he was not labelled on admission, this must be done now.

Drugs known as the premedication will have been prescribed by the doctor and are now given. Excess saliva and secretion of mucus from the bronchial tree are avoided by giving a drug which inhibits secretions, hyoscine being commonly used. Morphia or papaveretum (Omnopon) will make the patient sleepy and less aware of his surroundings. After these drugs have been given the patient should be quiet and he will go to sleep. When the theatre trolley arrives he should be lifted gently on to it with the minimum of disturbance and a nurse accompanies him to the theatre.

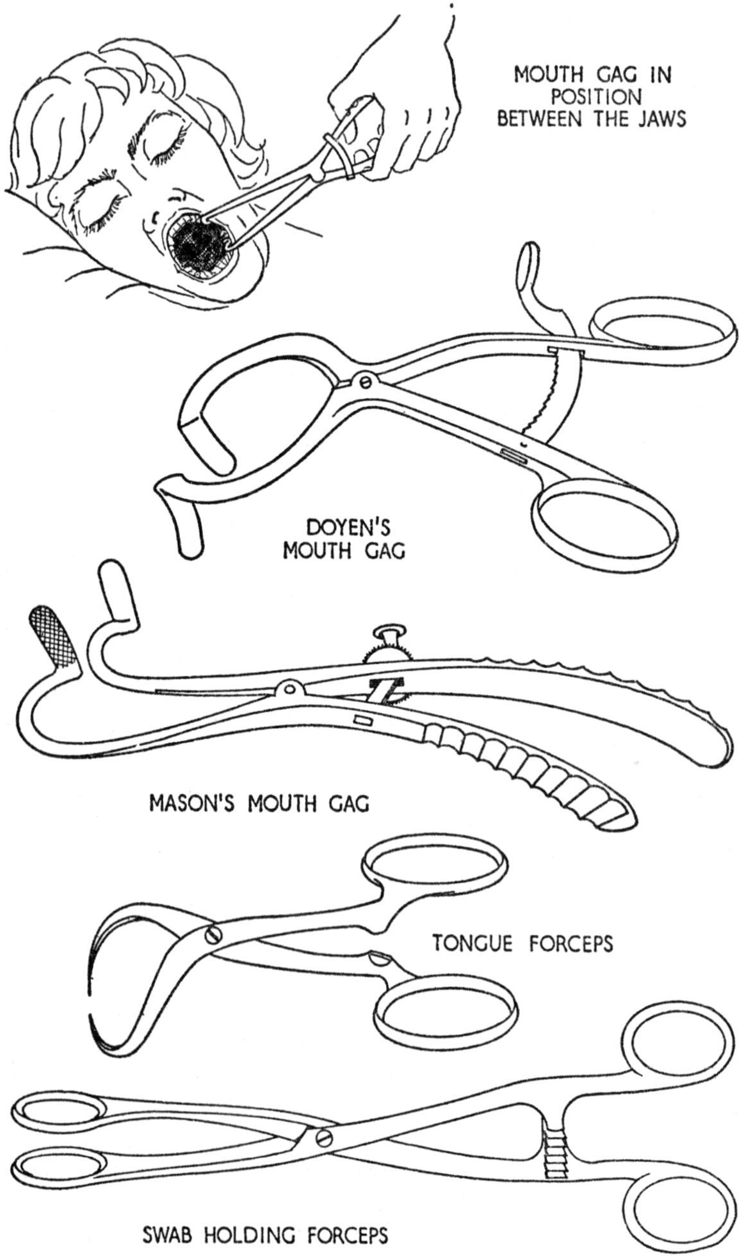

MOUTH GAG IN
POSITION
BETWEEN THE JAWS

DOYEN'S
MOUTH GAG

MASON'S MOUTH GAG

TONGUE FORCEPS

SWAB HOLDING FORCEPS

FIG. 56 Post-anaesthetic instruments

Nurse takes with her the patient's notes and X-rays and she also takes a tray of instruments ready for the return journey. These consist of a mouth gag, tongue forceps, swabholding forceps together with a vomit bowl and cloth.

Nurse stays with the patient while he is anaesthetized and if time permits she remains in the theatre during the operation.

Preparation for Return

In the ward the patient's bed is prepared for his return. Clean bed linen is used and the top bedclothes are folded into a pack which can be lifted to cover the patient quickly. Pillows are removed and the top of the bed protected. The surgeon may request that the bed be warmed. Any special apparatus, such as suction, is prepared, and a chart for the pulse is made ready. Bed blocks are brought to the bed. This should all be done as soon as the patient has left the ward so that if an emergency arises and he returns sooner than expected his bed is ready.

Immediate Care

A nurse from the ward goes to collect the patient from the theatre. She receives any instructions about his care from the surgeon and obtains permission from the anaesthetist to take the patient. During the journey to the ward the nurse is at the head of the trolley, watching the patient carefully and holding the jaw forward as in Fig. 58. She has with her the tray of instruments which went to the theatre and when she reaches the ward this tray is put on the locker. The patient is lifted gently into bed, and placed either on his side or on his back with the head turned to one side. After major surgery it may be advisable to leave the stretcher canvas under the patient until his general condition has improved. Any drainage tubes are inspected to see that they are not obstructed and connected to the suction apparatus as ordered. If intravenous fluid is being given the bottle is hung on the stand by the bedside and nurse ensures the fluid is running properly at the desired rate.

Care of Airway

With modern anaesthesia most patients recover consciousness soon after their return, indeed, some do so before getting back to the ward. A nurse stays with the patient until he is conscious and she has certain responsibilities during this time. The

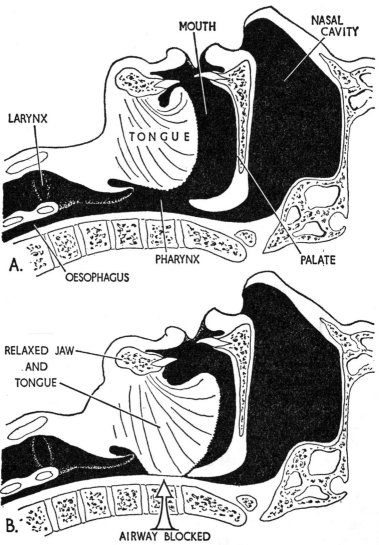

FIG. 57 How the tongue falls back

most important duty is to make sure that air is entering the lungs. The air passages may become blocked with mucus or vomit, or the tongue may slip back into the throat. If this happens, the patient's colour will change and he will become

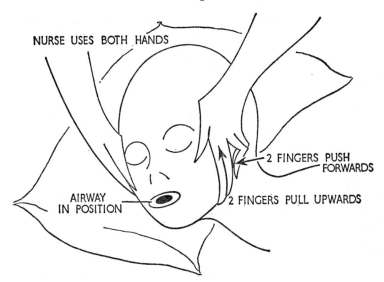

NURSE USES BOTH HANDS

2 FINGERS PUSH FORWARDS

AIRWAY IN POSITION

2 FINGERS PULL UPWARDS

FIG. 58 Holding the jaw forward

cyanosed very quickly. Nurse should open the patient's mouth, using the mouth gag to separate the jaws if necessary and she will then be able to see the cause of the obstruction. If the tongue has slipped back it should be brought forward. Mucus and fluid are mopped out, using moist gauze swabs on sponge-holding forceps and usually with these measures the patient's colour will return to normal. If it does not, however, no time should be lost before help is summoned.

Other Observations

The pulse should be counted and recorded every 15 minutes. Any change in rate or rhythm should be reported at once. The patient's appearance should also be watched carefully. Pallor and sweating are danger signs and must not go unobserved or unreported.

Recovery of consciousness is shown by the patient coughing and spitting out his airway. He opens his eyes and makes an attempt to move; speech is difficult, but he may try to say something. He should be given one pillow and will go to sleep for a short time; observations will be continued, though it is no longer necessary for a nurse to remain closely at the bedside.

With further recovery to consciousness another pillow may be given and patients appreciate having the face and hands sponged. A mouth wash may be given or sips of water if allowed, and dentures may be replaced. There may be pain and restlessness; these are controlled by giving the analgesic which will have been ordered by the doctor. Depending on the severity of the operation and the patient's condition, he will be arranged as soon as possible in the position in which he will be nursed and the theatre gown will be exchanged for his own night clothes.

The subsequent care of this patient now depends on what operation has been performed. If the operation was removal of the appendix (appendicectomy), with a clean stitched wound, the post-operative care should be straightforward as follows:

Diet

As soon as the patient can tolerate it, food should be given, in small quantities at first. By the third day after the operation a normal diet should be enjoyed.

Cleanliness

Depending on the patients age and general condition, he may need help with washing and a bed bath for a time after his operation. As soon as he is able to walk to the bathroom he will be able to complete his own toilet and may have a general bath provided that the dressing is waterproof.

Exercises

On the day after operation the patient will sit out whilst his bed is made. He will be encouraged both by the nurse and the physiotherapist to do his breathing and leg exercises. As soon as possible he will be helped to walk to the lavatory and bathroom.

Bowels

With early ambulation and eating a normal diet the patient often has a bowel action in the normal way, if not, glycerine suppositories may be given. After abdominal and pelvic operations the patient often suffers a good deal of pain and discomfort due to the presence of air in the intestines. This flatulence may be relieved by the passing of a flatus tube (see page 118) or a covered hot water bottle may be applied to the abdomen.

Records

A record of the temperature and pulse should be kept and any change in either must be reported.

Pain

A certain amount of discomfort is felt for twenty-four hours after operation and an analgesic will be ordered to relieve this. Subsequently the patient should feel very well and be free from pain.

Discharge

If the patients condition is satisfactory and his home conditions are good he may be discharged on the fourth day. Arrangements are made for the home nurse to remove his stitches, or he may return to the hospital for this to be done.

Wound

A clean stitched wound is left covered and undisturbed until the stitches are removed between the eighth and twelfth day.

Removal of Stitches

The requirements for this procedure must be sterile and may be supplied to the ward ready for use. Nurse will need:

    A few wool and gauze swabs
    A gallipot of spirit
    Dissecting forceps and stitch scissors (or stitch cutter)

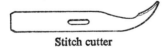

Stitch cutter

    Towels
    Paper bag for dirty dressings
    Receiver for used instruments
    Strapping or plastic spray

The patient is told what is about to happen and he is assured that the discomfort will be minimal. He is arranged on his bed or a couch lying on his back with one pillow under his head. He is covered except for the area round the wound.

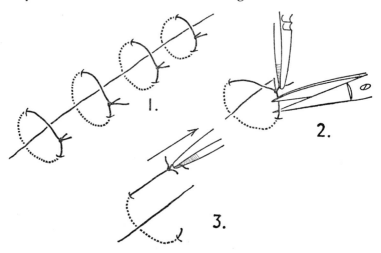

FIG. 59 Removing separate stitches

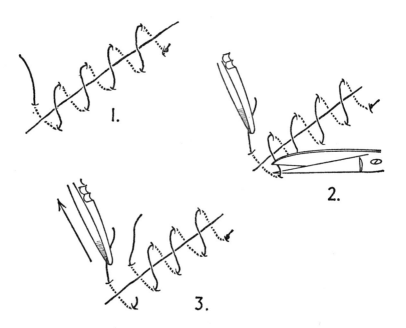

FIG. 60 Removing continuous suture

Nurse washes her hands thoroughly and dries them. A towel is laid over the patient as near the wound as possible. The strapping covering the wound is removed so that the stitches are exposed. If necessary the suture line is cleaned using swabs held in forceps. There may be either a line of separate stitches or one continuous suture. To remove the former, the knot of the stitch is held with dissecting forceps and gently lifted away from the skin. The stitch is snipped here and withdrawn from the other side of the wound so that the part of the suture which has been outside is not drawn through the wound. A continuous suture is removed in a similar manner snipping the stitch at one end and gently pulling it out from the other end.

A dry dressing may be applied for a few days to prevent the patient's clothing rubbing on the new scar.

Return to Work

A certain amount of time should elapse before the patient resumes work. Most patients have seven to ten days at home after the stitches have been removed, so that the total time away is between two and three weeks. He is instructed to visit his general practitioner and may be asked to attend the follow-up clinic in the 'Out Patients' Department.

CHAPTER 19

THE PATIENT WITH A FRACTURE

The body has a jointed bony framework, the skeleton. Some animals, like crabs, keep their skeletons on the outside, people keep theirs on the inside and clothe it in muscle and skin. Parts of the skeleton are also adapted to give protection to underlying organs; the skull protects the brain, the rib cage protects the heart and lungs. The bones are made of soft gristle stiffened with the salts of calcium and phosphorus just as aprons are made of soft linen stiffened with starch. It is possible to tie a bone into a knot by soaking it in acid until the salts have dissolved away, and all that is left is a soft pliable 'bone' of fibrous tissue. The first salts are deposited in a baby's bones before it is born, as will be seen in the X-ray of a pregnant woman. After this more and more salts are needed as the bones gradually harden and then grow until they reach adult size. There are four factors necessary for this purpose:

Calcium
Phosphorus ⎫ in the diet
Vitamin D ⎭

Parathormone, a hormone from the parathyroid gland.

Every day of life some part of the structure of the bones is being renewed, and if a bone is broken the normal replacement rate is increased as fresh bone is laid down to make the broken bone as strong as before.

Fractures

A bone may be broken or fractured (they mean the same thing) either directly or indirectly. Being thrown off a motor bicycle when not wearing a crash helmet may result in a fractured skull (direct fracture), but falling from a height on to the feet may be sufficient to fracture the skull as the result of the force passing through the body (indirect fracture). There are several different ways of describing the way in which a bone has broken. A SIMPLE FRACTURE is one in which the bone has broken across. A COMPLICATED FRACTURE is one involving other structures such as blood vessels or nerves. A COMPOUND FRACTURE is one in which the bone comes in contact with the air, either because the bone ends poke through the skin or because there is a wound from the surface down to the bone. This is dangerous because infection may enter the bone.

Care and Treatment of a Patient with a Fractured Limb

When a bone has been broken those with the victim suspect that this has happened because he complains of pain and cannot use the affected limb. They may also notice that it is lying in an unnatural position. They usually give first aid treatment which consists of splinting the limb, the best splint available being the patient's own body. If the 'bad' leg is tied to the 'good' leg and the 'bad' arm to the chest this will hold most fractures in position. When the patient reaches hospital the doctor will order drugs for the relief of pain and check the diagnosis by X-ray.

Following serious accident or injury there is not only the local condition but a general reaction of all the body tissues. This reaction is called 'shock'. There is a decrease in the volume of the circulating blood and the patient is cold and clammy with a low blood pressure. The treatment is to give an analgesic to relieve pain, and to increase the amount of circulating blood by giving fluid directly into the veins. To help keep the blood in the vital centres of heart and brain the foot of the bed may be raised on blocks and extra oxygen may help the blood that *is* circulating to carry all it can. The ward nurses will therefore prepare the following:

An admission bed with one pillow.

Fracture boards and a cradle if a lower limb is involved.

An extra drawsheet and waterproof sheeting to place under the limb.

Bed elevator.

Oxygen.

Requirements for giving an intravenous infusion.

Requirements for giving injections of analgesics (these are drugs for the relief of pain).

Requirements for giving injections of serum or toxoid.

Apparatus for recording the patient's temperature, pulse, respirations and blood pressure with the necessary charts.

Sandbags to act as temporary supports.

Waterproof covered pillows if the patient comes *from* the plaster room.

Reduction or Setting

After the patient has been admitted to the ward and had his initial treatment for shock the nurses will observe and report on his condition until the doctor decides that it is time for the bone to be set. During this waiting period the patient is moved as little as possible and no attempt is made to remove clothing or shave and cleanse the limb as this can be done in the theatre. Nothing should be given by mouth. The bone is then set. This means placing the bone ends as nearly as possible back into the correct position. A general anaesthetic is almost always given and the doctor either pulls the bone into position from outside (checking with X-rays) which is called CLOSED REDUCTION, or operates on the patient and manipulates the bone ends from inside which is called OPEN REDUCTION. Once the bone ends are in the right position they are held there (this is called immobilization) whilst the bone heals. They may be held from the inside with plates and screws like those in Fig. 61 or from the outside with a splint. Most patients have plaster of Paris splints, and it is usual for the joint above the fracture and the joint below the fracture to be immobilized.

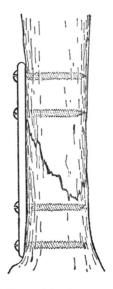

FIG. 61 Internal fixation of a fracture

When the patient's bone has been set and immobilized he returns to the ward. He is given normal post-operative care as for any patient, with special care to his injured limb.

Care of the Patient in Plaster

Immediate. Whilst a plaster is wet great care must be taken to see that it is not dented on the outside. If this happens the inner surface may be pushed in and cause damage to the underlying skin. Thus a wet plaster should always be handled with the flat of the hand, never the finger tips, and should only be placed on soft protected surfaces. A waterproof covered pillow is a sensible thing to use. Air should be allowed to circulate freely round a wet plaster so that it may dry slowly, quick drying may cause cracks.

Later. The nurse should pay attention at all times to the fingers and toes of the limb in plaster. These should always be:

> Warm.
> Pink.
> Mobile.

If the fingers or toes become cold, swollen, blue, or the patient is unable to move them, the nurse should inform sister immediately as this may mean there is obstruction to the blood or nerve supply owing to the pressure of the plaster. Sister may try for a short time to see whether the swelling will decrease if the limb is raised, but she will soon send for the doctor if there is no improvement, as the plaster may have to be cut. This is so important that all good nurses automatically look at toes and fingers as they go to the bedside and develop a reflex of:

> Look (are they pink?)
> Touch (are they warm?)
> Question (can the patient move them?)

The nurse should also take note of the patient's complaints about the plaster. PAIN SHOULD NEVER BE DISREGARDED especially if the patient can point to the place with one finger, as this often means that there is a sore under the plaster. If a sore is suspected, the patient's temperature is taken as a rise in temperature may indicate the presence of inflammation. Another check is to feel the plaster over the spot, if it is warm there may be a sore underneath and the doctor should be told. Patients sometimes try to ease discomfort by pushing cotton wool down their plasters. This is foolish as it will form lumps and make

M

the plaster even more uncomfortable. Trimming the top of the plaster may help but it should only be done by experts. In hot weather the patient may appreciate cool air from a hair dryer inside his plaster!

Care of the Patient in Traction

Sometimes patients have their limbs placed in special splints as shown in Figs. 62, 63 and 64. Nurses should find out whether

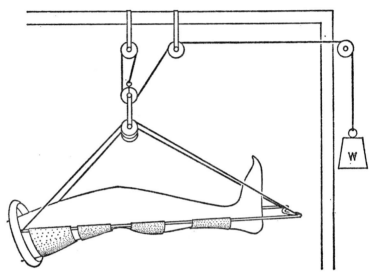

FIG. 62 Limb supported in a Thomas splint
Note: This patient is *not* in traction; the *weight* is supporting the splint

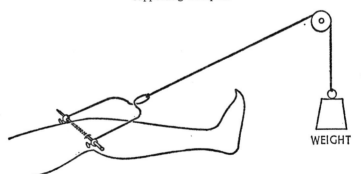

FIG. 63 Skeletal traction. (*Note:* Supporting splint not shown.)

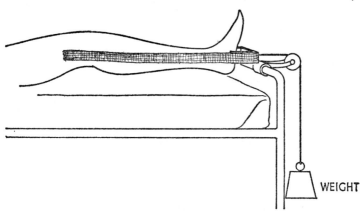

FIG. 64 Skin traction (bandages not shown)

the splint is simply supporting the limb or whether part of the limb is being pulled upon at the same time. The two can be distinguished by an inspection of the weights at the foot of the bed. If the weight is actually attached to the limb by means of a cord fastened to a metal bar through the limb, or to strapping placed on each side of the limb, then the patient is on 'traction'. If this is so it is particularly important that the weights hang freely and are not allowed to rest on the floor or be lifted on to the bed. If they do they will not be pulling on the bone as the doctor ordered.

There are certain places where the skin is likely to become sore and these should be checked daily and any potential soreness reported.

It is necessary to check daily:
under the ring of the splint, ⎫
under the patient's heel, ⎬ for soreness.
round the patient's ankle, ⎭
that the slings are secure,
that there is a pad under the knee,
that the patient is warm and protected from draughts.

General Care and Prevention of Complications

Whether the patient is in plaster or in a special splint the general rule is IMMOBILIZE THE LIMB AND MOBILIZE THE PATIENT. Most of the complications arise from the fact that the patient is sitting in bed, and they include:

Chest infection
Urinary infection
Bedsores
Venous thrombosis
Stiffness of the muscles and joints.

Position

The patient must sit up in bed as much as possible to help his breathing, being laid flat once a day to prevent stiffness of the hip.

Diet

His diet should be a full one with plenty of protein and extra calcium, phosphorus and Vitamin D to help his bone to heal rapidly and his muscle tone to remain good. He must drink plenty of fluid to help prevent stagnation of urine which may result in stone formation or infection.

Pressure Areas

As he is sitting very much in one position his pressure areas need constant attention. He should lift himself up and move about in bed as much as possible and a sorbo ring may be helpful. The most uncomfortable place apart from his sacral area is often the heel of the 'good' leg and the elbow of the arm nearest his locker which he leans on often.

Movement

The physiotherapist and the nurses must encourage the patient to move freely and carry out all his exercises. These include not only those for the muscles of the limb in splint or plaster but all the other joints or muscles of the body which he will later need to use when he returns to normal living. In exercising the lower limb it is very important to keep the ankle mobile and prevent 'foot drop' and to maintain the tone of the quadriceps, the muscles in the front of the thigh. This movement of the muscles of the legs also helps to prevent venous thrombosis. Thus the patient is encouraged to do most things for himself such as washing, lifting on and off bedpans, managing his meal trays and so forth.

Management

The fracture may take many weeks to heal and the patient must be given plenty to keep him occupied during this time. Many of the patients are young and apart from their fractures are soon feeling well. Nurses working on a fracture ward should be careful to maintain a professional attitude to their patients at all times or they may perhaps unwittingly provoke a situation in which it becomes difficult for a patient to maintain his self-control. On the other hand, a reasonably permissive attitude should be adopted towards all the equipment which the patient collects when he is doing his occupational therapy.

As his fracture heals he will gradually start more strenuous exercises and if it is a fracture of a lower limb he will start learning to walk once more. His first steps are usually taken in a walking machine and then he will graduate to crutches. Walking on crutches starts long before the patient is allowed to take any weight on his limb. Eventually he will be discharged as fit to return to his work or to be sent to a rehabilitation centre to work until he is fit to return to his normal job.

Special Care of Elderly Patients with Fractures

In old age the bones are so brittle that elderly patients may fracture a bone simply by tripping over the mat. A common fracture is that of the neck of the femur. As old people die of the complications rather than the fracture, the most important thing is to fix the fracture quickly so that the patient may be got out of bed as soon as possible. When they are admitted they are laid in bed with the limb between sandbags. As soon as possible they are taken to the theatre and the doctor, after cutting the skin, will pass a special nail through the fractured bone to hold it in place. (Fig. 65).

Back in the ward these patients present many nursing problems.

Mental State

Their mental state may be very confused. Once an elderly person is removed from her familiar home and her ordered routine she may become as unhappy as a child in the same circumstances. Any familiar links with home and normal life should be preserved if possible. The patient may be comforted by her own shawl, her

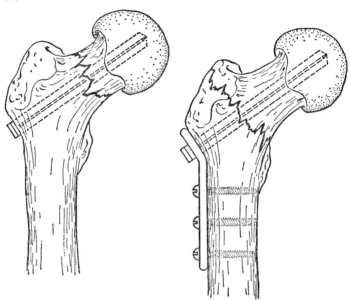

FIG. 65 Special nails used to hold a fractured neck of femur

own bedsocks and, perhaps, her own cup. Her relatives should be allowed to visit frequently even if they only sit quietly with the patient.

Physical State

The physical complications can be avoided if the patient's position can be changed easily and a good circulation maintained. If the patient is helped out of bed as soon as possible after operation this will reduce the chance of pressure sores, help prevent chest infection and, by increasing the circulation, will reduce the risk of venous thrombosis. The patient starts walking in the walking machine and after about six weeks she may start bearing weight on her leg. In due course she will be ready to go home and all the arrangements will have to be made for her.

Thus there are three important factors in the healing of a fracture, all of which are necessary for a successful outcome. The first is the skill of the surgeon who 'sets' the fracture and places the broken bone ends in a good position. Secondly, the skill of the nurse in keeping the limb in the position that the surgeon orders whilst preventing any complications from affecting the patient. Thirdly, the power of the patient's bone cells to grow and replace themselves which is the only thing which makes the healing of a fracture possible, and, in addition, the patience and co-operation of the patient throughout the long wearisome weeks of waiting and exercising until his limb is ready for use once more.

FURTHER READING

Nash, *Principles of Surgery and Surgical Nursing (Chapter 46).* Edward Arnold.

CHAPTER 20

THE NURSE AND THE
UNCONSCIOUS PATIENT

Communications are important. In living creatures they are the means by which the individual makes contact with everything outside, and everything outside makes contact with him.

The centre of the body's system of communications is the brain. The spinal cord is an important continuation of the brain. Nerve fibres pass to and from the brain via the spinal cord. The brain can be likened to a main telephone exchange, the spinal cord to a sub-exchange, and the nerve fibres to telephone wires. The fibres are seldom found alone—they lie in pairs, or groups, rather like cables. These 'cables' are the nerves. Nerves are found in the skin, in every organ and every blood vessel. They bring in messages from the outside through the skin, the ears, the eyes, the nose and the mouth to depots either in the spinal cord or in the brain. These depots either relay messages to other nerves or deal with them.

Man possesses a most highly-developed communications system. He has the powers of thinking, feeling and knowing, and his actions are governed accordingly. Very complex situations can be tackled by the 'higher centres' found in the cerebral cortex of the brain. The cerebral cortex consists of large areas of nerve cells.

The cerebral cortex, or rind of grey matter, is the outer part of the greater brain (cerebrum) and is protected by three coverings (meninges) under the skull bones. Deep within the brain substance other collections of nerve cells are found. These are called the basal ganglia.

The lower parts of the brain (*medulla and pons*), are responsible for simple reflexes—salivation on smelling something delectable, or blinking when a fleck of dust is near the eye. The centres controlling blood pressure and breathing are in the medulla.

Beneath the greater brain lies the *lesser brain* (*cerebellum*). Information of the body's positions is collected here. The cerebellum carries out some of the orders given by the cerebrum in a

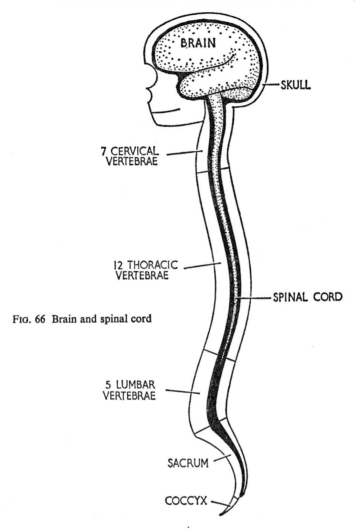

FIG. 66 Brain and spinal cord

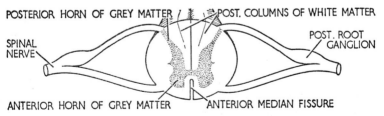

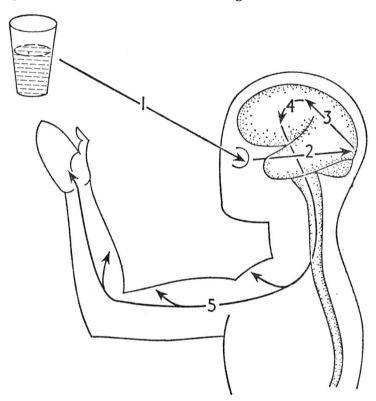

FIG. 67 Outside message results in action

smooth and efficient manner. Some of the messages entering the
cerebellum can be dealt with without them rising to consciousness, *i.e.*, without them going to the cerebrum.

The brain can be said to be mapped out into AREAS, each
area being responsible for a definite function. The posterior area
receives impressions from the eyes.

The meninges completely cover the whole surface of the brain
and spinal cord. A watery fluid—cerebro-spinal fluid—circu-
lates between the meninges. It acts as a buffer and it protects
the brain and spinal cord from jolts and jars.

It will be noticed, therefore, that the body's most important
functions are safeguarded by the centres lying deep within the
skull—as well protected as any part can be.

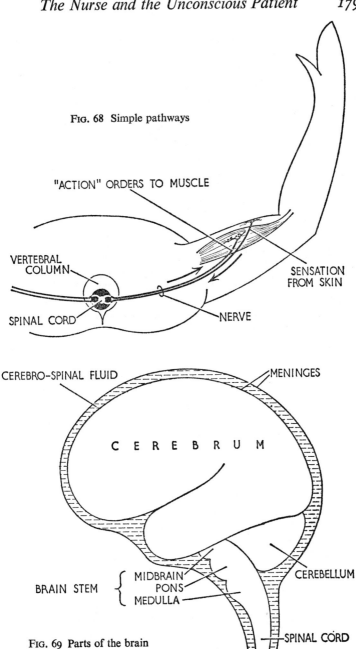

FIG. 68 Simple pathways

"ACTION" ORDERS TO MUSCLE

VERTEBRAL COLUMN

SENSATION FROM SKIN

SPINAL CORD

NERVE

CEREBRO-SPINAL FLUID

MENINGES

C E R E B R U M

MIDBRAIN
PONS
MEDULLA

BRAIN STEM

CEREBELLUM

SPINAL CORD

FIG. 69 Parts of the brain

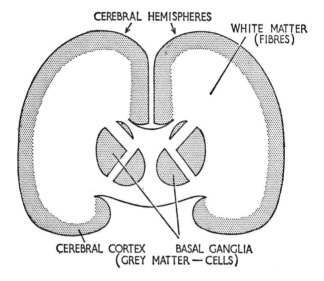

FIG. 70 Section through brain showing grey and white matter

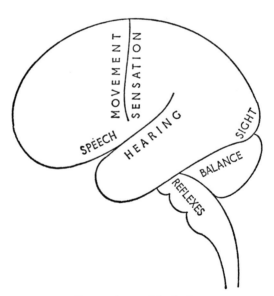

FIG. 71 Areas of the brain

Unconsciousness

When a person does not respond to stimuli and cannot be roused, he is said to be unconscious. Sometimes the phrase 'in coma' is used.

Causes of Unconsciousness

Anaesthetic unconsciousness. A general anaesthetic renders a patient unconscious. The depth of it is very carefully controlled by the anaesthetist so that the surgeon can operate in the best possible way. After the operation the patient requires constant observation until consciousness is regained.

Traumatic unconsciousness. An increasing number of patients are found in the general wards of many hospitals with 'traumatic unconsciousness'. This is often the result of accidents in fast-moving traffic, or of falling from a height, or of blows on the head. When force is applied to the head the brain inside the skull is jarred, and intra-cranial shock (concussion) may result. Concussion may last from a few minutes to several days or weeks, and may be accompanied by severe injuries to the scalp and skull. Many patients require the suturing of superficial wounds. Few of them need major surgery involving lengthy operations, but some patients will need to go to the operating theatre for the relief of compression. Compression may be caused by a depressed fracture of the skull, or the formation of a blood clot beneath the skull bones.

Other Causes of Unconsciousness are:

(a) Disturbances in the circulation of blood in the brain, such as clotting or haemorrhage or diminution of blood supply which causes fainting.

(b) Pressure within the skull which may be caused by tumours of the brain, inflammation of the coverings (meningitis), or of the brain itself (encephalitis).

(c) Poisoning by drugs or gases.

(d) Alterations in blood chemistry, as with the excessive intake of alcohol, or in the condition of diabetes mellitus.

In all these instances communications are lost; the patient is unconscious.

Observation

Keen observation of every unconscious patient is essential.

Information obtained by the nurse will help the doctor to assess the actual condition of the patient. Improvement is noted, deterioration can be seen, and complications will be indicated. An accurate assessment of the whole patient is necessary, as on this depends the management of the patient.

On admission the nurse must take note of the general appearance of the patient, especially his colour. The nose, and ears and mouth are looked into for bleeding or discharge of fluid. Any difference felt when handling the limbs may suggest paralysis. Comment must be made on the condition of the skin. It is dry in diabetic coma, moist in insulin coma, and cold and clammy in shock. Sometimes marks of needle punctures, where drugs have been injected, can be seen. Smelling the breath may indicate the consumption of alcohol. The odour of acetone can be detected in diabetic coma.

Recording of observations. The recording of observations on a chart is started, and at intervals, varying from $\frac{1}{4}$ hour to 4 hours (chosen by the doctor) they are written down. The temperature, pulse and respiration rates and blood pressure are noted. A rising temperature may indicate damage to the brain stem or part of the basal ganglia, *e.g.*, the hypothalamus. The rate and volume of the pulse is required, also the rate, regularity and depth of the respirations.

A note should be made of response to stimuli, *i.e.*, opening the eyes on being asked, rousing on being called by name or on being moved, or on pressing above the eyes. A powerful 'George!' may bring about a response, whereas a delicate 'Mr England?' may not!

The state of the pupils, whether equal, dilated or contracted, and if they respond to light, are to be recorded. A spare column for other remarks is useful on the chart. Terms which are clearly understood by all should be used, and words like 'semi-conscious' and 'semi-comatose' are better avoided. Corneal reflexes are said to be absent if blinking does not occur when the cornea of the eye is gently touched with a fine strand of cotton wool.

The fact that the doctor relies on the nurse to make a clear picture of all the information cannot be stressed too much. Prompt reporting of accurate observations can provide diagnostic clues of immense value to the doctor, and ensures that urgent treatment can be given if necessary.

The nursing care of an unconscious patient can be directed along three main ways—the keeping of a clear airway, the providing of fluids and food and the prevention of complications.

The Keeping of a Clear Airway. The airway is the nurse's first concern. Dentures must be removed and all obstructions must be cleared without delay otherwise cyanosis and death will occur. A collection of mucus and saliva, a regurgitation of stomach contents or bleeding from the head and neck may block the air passages. Elevation of the foot of the bed for about forty-five centimetres helps to drain mucus and saliva out of the mouth.

Wherever possible the semi-prone position is used. A pillow is placed under the sheet, behind the back, and the upper leg if placed over the lower leg, helps to keep the position. If the patient is nursed on his back the tongue may fall back and obstruct the air passages.

The air passages may have to be cleared with suction. An electric sucker with a fairly stiff catheter (a small-sized Tiemann's catheter for instance) is the most satisfactory. With the help of a light, the pharynx may also be cleared, but this is generally the duty of a state registered nurse. Oxygen may be administered when the air passages are clear.

Even though a good position has been kept, and suction applied diligently, it may be necessary to do more. A cuffed endotracheal tube, inserted through the nose, into the trachea, gives a clear air passageway. A more permanent method is achieved by making an opening into the trachea with a scalpel, and then inserting a tracheostomy tube.

Throughout the whole period of unconsciousness, because normal secretions tend to accumulate, and the patient's reflexes are depressed, constant clearing of the air passages is essential, whatever aids are being employed.

The Providing of Fluids and Food. As the unconscious patient cannot swallow, nothing can be given by mouth. Efforts must be made, therefore, to maintain a food intake in other ways to avoid using the patient's body reserves. If there has been a considerable loss of fluid from the body, it may be necessary to give fluids by the intravenous route until a balance is restored. When food and fluids are needed over a long period, feeding through a tube passed into the stomach is a better method. As there is no cough reflex, the nurse must be especially careful when passing the tube. A diet can be prepared from milk, and proprietary protein and other substances, providing from 1800 to 2500 Calories a day, sufficient to nourish the patient. Water can be given freely, and dehydration is prevented. The fluid intake is recorded accurately on the patient's fluid balance chart.

Prevention of Complications. The maintenance of a clear airway saves the patient from asphyxia, and from broncho-pneumonia, by aspiration of vomit or mucus; fluid replacement avoids dehydration, and gastric intubation provides a satisfactory method of feeding, but other nursing problems remain. The unconscious patient not only requires the basic nursing care given to an ill patient, but is also dependent for his very survival on skilful nursing measures to prevent complications. Infection must be avoided at all costs.

Toxaemia from Pressure Sores. The majority of pressure sores are preventable, but if allowed to develop they will cause infection and become a serious threat to the patient's life. Cleanliness of the skin, and turning the patient from side to side every hour, day and night, is essential. As the patient is unable to receive any warnings of harmful pressure on the skin, hot water bottles, electric blankets and air rings must not be used.

Urinary Infections. The patient's condition is complicated by disturbances in bladder function. Retention, then retention with overflow, may occur, and the latter can be confused with incontinence of urine. Catheterization may be necessary and measures must be taken to avoid urinary infection. Antibiotics may be ordered by the doctor. Wherever possible the output of urine must be recorded on the chart.

Respiratory infections, especially broncho-pneumonia, arise quickly, but the lungs benefit from the two hourly turning of the patient, when the patient's position is changed.

Eyes. As well as the blinking reflex being absent in unconscious patients, sometimes the eyes are open, or partially open. Oily eye drops may be instilled. The surface of the eyeball could be damaged if the nurse was careless and let the bedclothes touch them.

Restlessness. Continuous supervision is necessary as the patient regains consciousness, because he may become restless. He may try to get out of bed, and may fall and injure himself in his confused state. He may be thirsty, or in pain, or wish to pass urine. The nurse must discover, if she can, the cause of this restlessness, and ask for assistance. Forceful restraint, without discovering the cause, will only make a restless patient more restless.

Unconscious Patients present a great challenge to nurses, calling for conscientious observations, and diligent and consistent nursing. Without first class nursing, many of these patients would die. The hard work involved is often extremely rewarding when an apparently hopeless patient recovers consciousness, and communications are satisfactorily restored.

FURTHER READING

Marshall, *Neurological Nursing*. Blackwell.
Ritchie, *Stroke, A Diary of Recovery*. Faber.

N

CHAPTER 21

THE NURSE AND THE PARALYSED PATIENT

Before attempting to understand paralysis it is important to understand how normal muscles act. The muscles which produce movement are placed like straps across the jointed framework of the body. They are made up of small elongated cells, all bound together by a fine, tough membrane called fascia. Those which move joints are usually attached to bones by strong, narrow tendons. Muscle cells are unique in the body in that they have the power to contract which makes them shorter. In order to do this they must, so to speak, be 'wired' to send and receive nerve impulses, as all movement in the body is started by electrical impulses passing along the nerves.

Information, also in the form of nerve impulses, is constantly being sent from all parts of the body through the spinal cord to the brain. Thus the brain is told which muscle cells are contracted, what position the joints are in, whether anything is touching the skin and many other things besides. In response to these incoming messages (sensory stimuli) the brain acts in two ways. Firstly, it always takes note of any new sensation and stores up the memory of it so that when a message is passed up again it can more easily be identified. Thus a message which passes up the first time as 'you have a pain in your right gluteal muscle' will later be received as 'you have sat on a drawing pin again'. Secondly, it sends messages back (motor impulses) to the appropriate muscles so that movement can be made.

If someone sits on a drawing pin it is usual to get up fairly quickly, and this means that the brain has had to send messages to many muscles telling them to contract and others to relax so that the person may stand up. However, in an emergency such as this, the brain may allow the spinal cord to deal directly with the situation, acting on its own through a 'short cut' (connector neurone) a split second before the brain receives the message. The person will find that he has risen to his feet before he knows it. This independent action of the spinal cord is called reflex action.

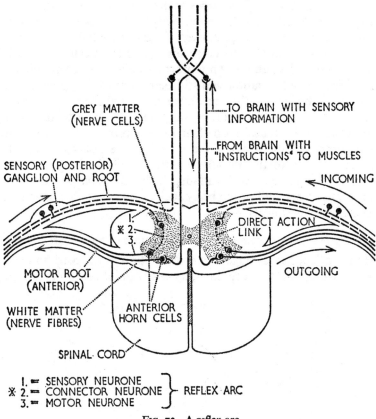

GREY MATTER
(NERVE CELLS)

......TO BRAIN WITH SENSORY
INFORMATION

.....FROM BRAIN WITH
"INSTRUCTIONS" TO MUSCLES

SENSORY (POSTERIOR)
GANGLION AND ROOT

INCOMING

DIRECT ACTION
LINK

1.
✗ 2.
3.

MOTOR ROOT
(ANTERIOR)

OUTGOING

WHITE MATTER
(NERVE FIBRES)

ANTERIOR
HORN CELLS

SPINAL CORD

1. = SENSORY NEURONE
✗ 2. = CONNECTOR NEURONE } REFLEX ARC
3. = MOTOR NEURONE

FIG. 72 A reflex arc

Two other points are worth noting; if messages are being
sent out from both the brain and the spinal cord, once the
first emergency is over, the impulses from the brain always take
priority and control those from the cord. It is also important
to remember that messages for the right side of the body come
from the left side of the brain and vice versa.

The Patient with Damage to One Side of the Brain

The brain can sustain one-sided damage in many ways, one of
the most common being a clot of blood blocking an artery supplying blood to the brain; rupture of a vessel in the brain is
another cause of damage. The damaged part of the brain will be

unable to send out any messages to the opposite side of the body, so the whole of one side of the body will be unable to move. The arm and leg will be powerless, the mouth will droop and the patient will be unable to close his eye. The affected side will feel numb to the patient as no information will be received from it. However, information will still be passed to the spinal cord, and once the cells in the cord have recovered from the general shock of damage to the brain, they may continue to send out impulses to the muscles on their own. Unfortunately, without the control of the brain, these messages are not very helpful, tending to make the muscles contract and the limbs stiffen. This type of paralysis with stiff muscles is called spastic paralysis. Paralysis of one half of the body such as occurs in this patient is known as hemiplegia.

The Patient with Damage to a Cross Section of the Spinal Cord

If the patient has damage to a cross section of the cord no messages will be able to reach the body at any point below the injury,

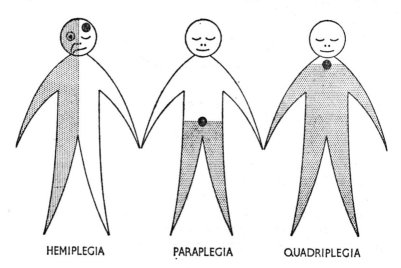

HEMIPLEGIA   PARAPLEGIA   QUADRIPLEGIA

FIG. 73 Types of paralysis

nor will any stimuli be able to reach the brain for interpretation. The patient will be unable to feel or move his limbs. He may, however, get strong muscle spasm caused by the direct action of the nerves of the spinal cord, but he has no control over these. Paralysis of both lower limbs is called paraplegia and that of all four limbs is called quadriplegia. Damage to a cross section of the cord often occurs in young people following a fracture of the spine due to an accident.

The Patient with Damage to the Motor Cells of the Cord

It is possible for some cells within the spinal cord to be damaged by disease whilst others continue to function. An example of this is when the motor relay cells in the spinal cord (the anterior horn) are attacked by the virus of poliomyelitis. (All motor nerve impulses whether from the brain or spinal cord pass through this point). If the anterior horn has been destroyed the affected nerve cells will be unable to pass on any messages. The muscles they supply will be completely limp and flaccid. The patient will still be able to feel his limbs because the route for incoming sensory stimuli will be undamaged and able to function. This patient may be paralysed anywhere, depending upon which sections of the cord have been attacked by the virus. A further complication may arise here, because if a muscle which bends a joint is left healthy, and its 'opposite number', the muscle which straightens the joint, is affected, the healthy muscle may pull the joint into an abnormal position.

Recovery

At first it is impossible to tell whether paralysis will be temporary or permanent. Even very badly damaged nerve cells may recover or have their function taken over by other cells. No nerve cell can ever be replaced, and after a certain time it will be possible to assess the amount of permanent damage. However, the extent of the paralysis must never be confused with the extent of the patient's disability. The loss of some muscles is far more disabling than others, depending upon whether other muscles can take over the work. Sometimes operations for stiffening joints or 'transplanting' muscles can be undertaken.

Care of a Patient with Hemiplegia

The reasons for hemiplegia are many and treatment may differ, but the nursing of this patient will be considered only in relation to his paralysis.

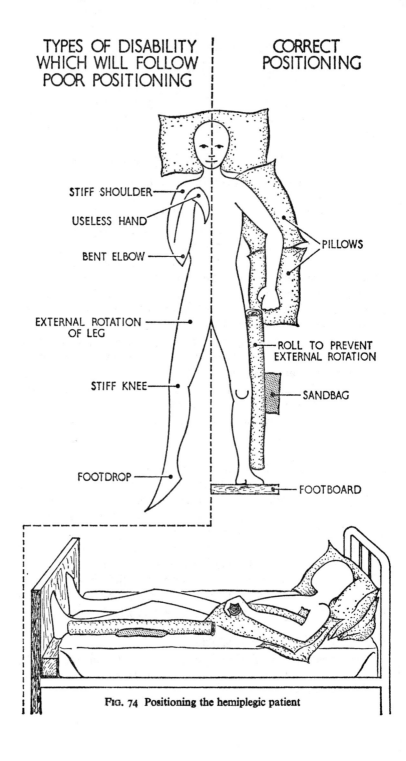

TYPES OF DISABILITY
WHICH WILL FOLLOW
POOR POSITIONING

CORRECT
POSITIONING

STIFF SHOULDER

USELESS HAND

BENT ELBOW

EXTERNAL ROTATION
OF LEG

STIFF KNEE

FOOTDROP

PILLOWS

ROLL TO PREVENT
EXTERNAL ROTATION

SANDBAG

FOOTBOARD

FIG. 74 Positioning the hemiplegic patient

Care of the Limbs

At first the chances of ultimate recovery are not known. The main function of the nurse is to act as 'caretaker' for the patient's joints and muscles whilst he is unable to move them himself. Should he never regain the use of his limbs the muscles will wither from disuse and the joints will stiffen, but at least proper care will have ensured that the limb still has some use. A stiff hand can perhaps be used as a holder for a spoon, a stiff foot as a pedestal for standing. If the patient does regain the use of his limbs he will want the joints to be 'well-oiled' and ready to be used by his feeble muscles as they slowly regain their strength. These results are obtained by careful attention to two points. Firstly, positioning of the limbs so that no muscle is overstretched and all joints are in the so-called neutral position. The neutral position is found by moving a joint to its fullest extent in either direction and positioning it between the two extremes. Secondly, by regular movement of all joints. At first these movements are passive, that is to say the patient takes no part, his limbs are moved for him. Later on he is able to move them if they are supported against the pull of gravity. Finally, he can move them on his own.

Positioning

The hand. This should be kept in the position shown in the drawing, the simplest method being to make a small plaster of Paris 'cock-up' splint which can be bandaged snugly into position. Each time the joints are moved the splint is removed and replaced.

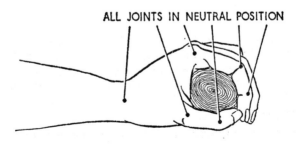

ALL JOINTS IN NEUTRAL POSITION

FIG. 75 Position of the hand

The foot. This is kept at an angle of 90 degrees as shown. The gap between the mattress and the foot board is helpful in preventing sore heels; but any type of foot board may be used and the leg may be supported by a pillow instead.

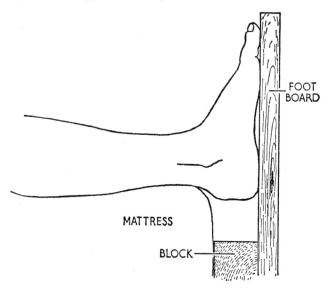

FIG. 76 Position of the foot

The shoulder. This is often forgotten. An angle of 45 degrees from the body is about right and it must be moved and repositioned frequently.

The hip. The whole leg must be prevented from rolling outwards. A long roll of blankets held in position by a sandbag is useful. No undue pressure should be applied when maintaining position, the weight of the bedclothes being taken by a bed cradle. The limbs are often very cold as the circulation is sluggish, and socks, mittens and shawls are all useful in providing warmth without weight. Both the nurse and the physiotherapist must play their part in giving passive exercises, but later on the physiotherapist will take the major part in giving supported exercises.

Care of the Skin

Skill is needed to prevent sores as the circulation is poor and the limbs are often a dead weight and, in addition, the patient is often incontinent of urine and faeces. He must be kept clean and dry and his position changed two hourly if sores are to be prevented. As soon as he can sit out of bed in a chair he should be helped to do so as this will be another possible change of position. Barrier creams may help to waterproof the skin and oil may keep it supple, but only regular turning of the patient will prevent sores.

Care of the Bladder and Bowels

The doctor will decide whether or not he wishes the patient to have a catheter in position all the time or if he is to be catheterised at intervals. A problem with an elderly, confused patient is to keep him from pulling the catheter out. The area round the catheter must be kept scrupulously clean, and an adequate fluid intake maintained to prevent urinary infection. The bowels should be regulated by means of regular enemas or suppositories.

Diet

The diet should have a good protein, iron and vitamin content but not too high a calorie value. The patient who cannot move himself and is dependent for his movements on the efforts of others should not be allowed to become too heavy. The greatest difficulty at first is chewing and swallowing, so soft foods are given. The patient must learn to take food into the 'good' or unparalysed side of his mouth, but at first the nurse discovers a great deal of 'lost' food when she carries out the regular cleansing of his paralysed cheek. As chewing improves he is able to take more solid food. An elderly patient's interest in food may be put to good account at this point, because his first move towards independence may be learning to feed himself.

Rehabilitation

Rehabilitation starts immediately after the onset of paralysis, and the nurse has prepared for it by her care of the limbs in the early stages. The other place where rehabilitation must start is in the patient's mind. Paralysis means dependence on others, rehabilitation means independence. A young patient, eager to get back to work, is easy to encourage to be self-supporting, but with an elderly, confused patient the battle is against apathy, loss of confidence, depression and loneliness. As has been mentioned before, the road to rehabilitation is often through the stomach. The first step to independence is to feed oneself. The patient may prefer to be fed, it is quicker and cleaner and far less effort. Then the battle of wits begins, for to every objection raised by the patient the nurse must have an answer. He cannot hold a spoon? She pads the handle until it is large enough for him to grasp. He cannot lift his arm? She arranges a sling from a runner in the ceiling to support it. He cannot eat meat with a spoon? She cuts it into small chunks which he may spear with a fork. His plate slips away? She puts it on a pad of foam rubber. His meat slips over the edge of the plate? She gives him a bowl instead. Her attitude must be warm and encouraging throughout and soon the visiting friends and relatives will have caught some of her enthusiasm.

This is the moment to discuss with them some of the special problems which will arise when the patient goes home. The British Red Cross Society publish an excellent booklet of gadgets, many of which a keen young grandson might make; the Occupational Therapy department will give help and support. Gradually the patients' interest in life returns as they practise to make themselves more self-supporting before discharge. Women like independence in the kitchen and though this may mean the use of such devices as a spike to hold a loaf whilst it is cut, one-handed independence can usually be achieved. Elderly gentlemen in the same way can learn to use such aids as nail brushes fixed to the wall to be used by the good hand. There may be a need for some alteration in the house apart from gadgets. For example, a new stair rail, perhaps a higher chair, an arm rest in the lavatory, or a lower bed may be needed and when these have been supplied the patient can return home happily.

Not all patients have happy or easily adaptable homes to go to; for them a different solution may be possible depending upon the social services available in the area. With a health visitor to supervise and co-ordinate the other services, an old lady or gentleman can live alone, drawing their old age pension supplemented by Supplementary Benefit. Their shopping, cooking and cleaning can be done by a home help, though in some areas a midday meal may come from 'Meals on Wheels' except at weekends. The district nurse, under orders from the doctor, will give such nursing attention as is needed, such as regular baths. Relatives, friends and neighbours will call in, the Vicar will visit and perhaps arrange a wheelchair ride to church. Alas, even this solution is not always possible and some must remain in hospital for the rest of their lives.

The Patient with Paraplegia

Although the basic principles of care are the same, the problems of the paraplegic patient are very different from those of the hemiplegic patient.

Management

Immediately after the accident or illness the patient is unable to comprehend what has happened to him. He may comment to the nurse that his limbs feel cold and numb, he may remark that he cannot move his leg, but the full implication of this is not apparent to him. As he reaches a fuller understanding of his plight his reactions range from anxiety to fear and finally despair. No nurse can follow her patient to the depths of despair. The fact of long months of rehabilitation or even permanent paralysis is something which the patient must face alone. All the nurse can do at this point is to see that all other worries are kept to a minimum. The medical social worker will explain the financial position, family and friends will visit, a message from 'the Boss' about a waiting job may encourage him. The nurse must be there at all times, calm, accepting and matter of fact in her attitude until the turning point is reached.

Every patient must, in the end, accept the fact that he must stop thinking about what he cannot do, and must start thinking about what he *can* do. After falling down a flight of stairs it is necessary to climb up again from the bottom, it is no good wishing to be at the top. Only when the patient starts thinking positively about his future can the nurse be of real use to him. Then she must watch for signs of returning independence and foster them. If his physical horizons are not very wide at the beginning she can always enlarge his mental ones—music, radio, television, news and books. All the time she is helping him prepare for the next step forward. She is the one to explain that all those exercises with Indian clubs are the basis of efficient wheelchair living and can stress the importance of strong shoulder muscles.

She explains the function of the long mirror as an aid to balance. She is the one who teaches the patient to dress himself, to swing in and out of bed and many other skills besides. She knows when to bully and when to help, when to come forward and when to withdraw.

Nursing Care

Care of limbs, skin, bladder and bowels are basically the same as for the hemiplegic patient. The patient may die if he develops chest infection, urinary infection or pressure sores, so these must be prevented. A bed like the one illustrated can be used and the patient is turned every two hours day and night. The special arrangement of the sorbo packs means that minimum pressure is applied to areas where the bones lie just under the skin. As

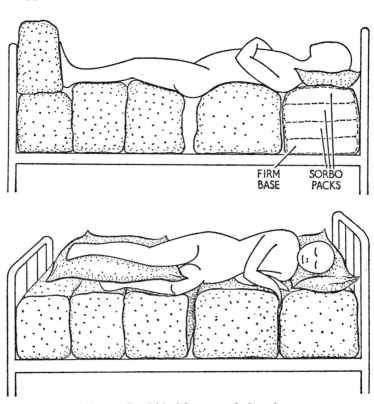

FIRM BASE   SORBO PACKS

FIG. 77 Special bed for a paraplegic patient

soon as possible the patient gets into his wheelchair where he must get used to his sitting position, gradually at first, and finally learn to balance himself steadily. He works hard to develop his shoulder muscles and learns to lift and turn himself. He has to lift up in his chair every half an hour to prevent pressure sores and must learn to examine himself for the early signs of soreness which he will never feel. As he may wish to travel away from home he may make use of an indwelling catheter and urine collecting bag. He must know not only how to pass the catheter, but also how to sterilize and care for the apparatus himself. He must know when an enema is necessary, and how to give himself one. He must realize the importance of drinking large quantities of fluid, as this prevents stagnation of urine with its attendant risks of infection.

Rehabilitation

The aim of rehabilitation is independence, to get back to work, to earn, to support a family. It may not be the same work as before the accident, the fireman may now be a draughtsman, the nurse a medical secretary, but it is useful paid employment. However, there is one group who do not wish to change their jobs, one group whose job has to be adapted to suit their changed circumstances, and these are housewives and mothers. It may mean changing the house for a bungalow, turning the steps into a ramp, having a higher oven, but it can be done. Even babies can be managed from a chair if the mother's apron has a large button to button the baby in the bottom of the apron whilst she takes both hands to her chair. Invalid cars promise even greater independence.

Thus it will be seen that many types and degrees of paralysis exist. The aim of the nurse is to encourage the patient towards as much independence as is possible for *him*. The actual recovery of the nerves is beyond the control of the patient, but the success of his own recovery depends entirely upon himself.

FURTHER READING

Bates & Pellow, *Horizontal Man* (*Story of a Polio Victim*). Longmans.

Marshall, *Two Lives*. Hutchinson.

Opie, *Over My Dead Body*. Methuen.

Wilkinson and Fisk, *Orthopaedic Nursing*. Faber.

CHAPTER 22

UNDERSTANDING THE TOXIC PATIENT

Man can be described as a warm-blooded animal. In spite of the wide variations in the temperature outside his body he keeps his body temperature constant. The normal body temperature is within the range 36° to 37·5°C. (97° to 99·5°F.). In health it is kept within this range because the body maintains a balance between heat produced and heat lost.

In temperate climates heat production depends chiefly on the burning up of food in the cells of the body, especially in the cells of the glands and the muscles. Heat loss depends on radiation, and on evaporation of sweat from the body. As the water evaporates from the body, heat is lost, as it gets taken up into the air. There is also a certain amount of heat lost from the lungs in respiration.

Fever

Fever, or pyrexia, is a sign that the temperature-regulating centre of the brain is disturbed. It can be disturbed by injury, or more commonly by infections which are due to:

(*a*) bacteria—for example in pneumonia

(*b*) viruses—for example in influenza

(*c*) protozoa—for example in malaria.

In fever the amount of heat produced is increased, and the amount of heat lost is decreased, therefore the balance is disturbed. When a part of the body is inflamed, *e.g.*, a whitlow develops on a finger, certain reactions occur. These reactions are protective, and are outward, visible signs of inward changes inside the body. There is heat, redness, pain, swelling and loss of function of the finger. Because they occur at the site of the inflammation, they are called LOCAL REACTIONS. The body as a whole tries to overcome the infection too, and the temperature rises. It may reach 39°C. (103°F.), or even higher. This is a GENERAL REACTION to the infection. Other effects of fever are headache, loss of appetite, disinclination to work or be energetic, feeling hot on a cold day, feeling cold on a hot day, or feeling both at the same time.

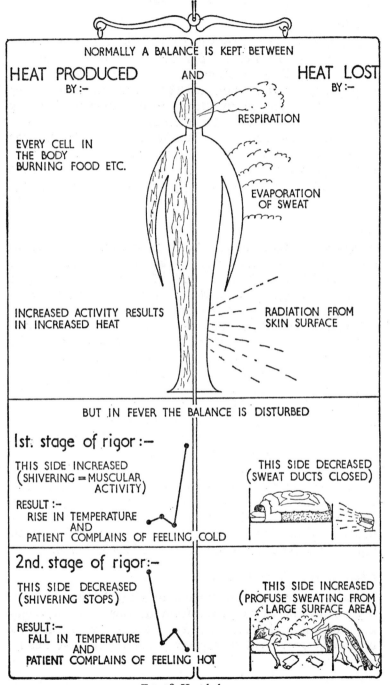

FIG. 78 Heat balance

The Body's Defence

In infections the number of white blood cells (leucocytes) in the circulating blood increases from the normal 7,000 to 8,000 in each cubic millimetre of blood, to something approaching 12,000 or 15,000, or even more. This is called leucocytosis. They increase in number in an attempt to overcome the invading bacteria which are causing the infection.

Sometimes the glands near the site of the infection become enlarged, *e.g.*, the lymphatic glands in the axilla (of the arm) when there is a whitlow on the finger. This shows that they are defending the part, making more lymphocytes, and filtering the bacteria.

Rigor

A rigor is a shivering attack. As the patient's temperature rises (rate of heat production being greater than the rate of heat loss) he shivers, and he complains of feeling cold. Shivering is an effort on the part of the muscles to produce heat. The temperature is rising because he is shivering. It is not because he feels cold that he is shivering. At the same time his skin is hot and dry, and he is not losing any moisture from it. The bedclothes are pulled up round his neck, and the patient still complains of feeling cold. After about half an hour the shivering stops and the temperature starts to fall. This is because the heat production in the muscles is less. The skin starts to sweat, increasing heat loss. The patient then says that he is hot, and the bedclothes are thrown off, allowing for more evaporation of sweat from the skin. This brings the temperature down.

This rapid rise of temperature, associated with shivering, and feeling cold, and followed by a fall in temperature, sweating and feeling hot, (a rigor) is caused by an influx of foreign protein into the bloodstream. It happens in malaria when the parasite liberates its offspring into the bloodstream. It is an unfavourable sign if it occurs during an intravenous infusion of blood.

Characteristic Temperatures

In many other diseases the temperature gradually rises, and then it gradually falls as the patient recovers. This occurs especially in pneumonia and in influenza. The shapes of the graphs made on the charts vary with the types of infections. They are a useful guide to the events occurring within the body. (Refer to drawings of charts of actual conditions).

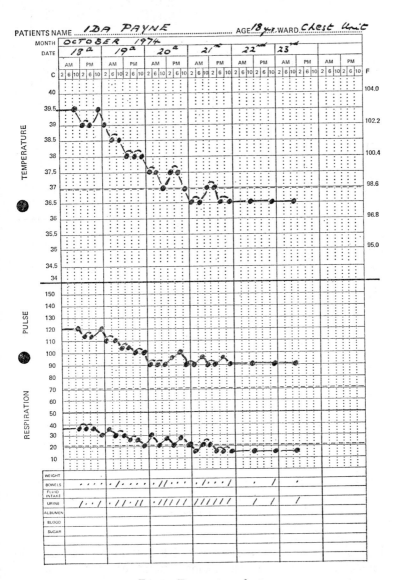

FIG. 79 Temperature chart

o

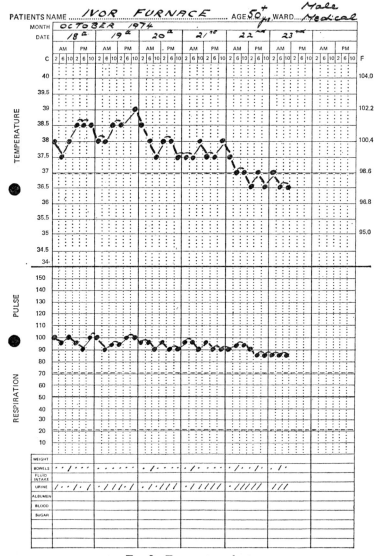

FIG. 80 Temperature chart

Types of Infection

Disease-producing bacteria are called pathogens, and are responsible for many diseases of man. Injurious effects of pathogenic bacteria on the body are due to the chemical substances

they release during their growth, or on their breakdown after they die. These substances are called TOXINS. In causing disease toxins follow specific patterns. The tubercle bacillus causes tuberculosis only—it cannot cause diphtheria. Some organisms, *e.g.*, staphylococcus, can cause disease in the lungs—pneumonia, and also in bones—osteomyelitis. On the other hand pneumonia can be caused by many other organisms. Only by much learning can the differences be understood and appreciated.

(*a*) *Streptococcal Infection.* The cause of pain on swallowing, a symptom of a sore throat, may be the haemolytic streptococcus, a type of bacteria. The tonsils, the lymphatic glands in the throat, often become infected, and this situation may be the herald of scarlet fever, or some other disease. The patient has a rash in scarlet fever, but the infection is not in the skin. The throat carries the infection and droplets from it may infect other people. Streptococci do not usually invade the whole body. They tend to stay around the tonsils, and they send out their poisonous toxins into the bloodstream. The toxins make the rash. To combat the toxins the patient makes his own specific ANTITOXINS to neutralize them. These antitoxins are retained even when the rash has gone and the disease is over. They protect the person from a second attack of scarlet fever, but he may still get streptococcal sore throats, and pass them on. (It is obvious from this that nurses and doctors should not be on duty with sore throats, unless it has been proved that they are not spreading disease by droplet transmission).

(*b*) *Other Infections.* Sometimes the bacteria are more subtle. In diphtheria, the organisms also live in the throat, and send out toxins, but there is no rash. Instead of causing a rash, they may damage the heart muscle. Specially prepared antitoxin is given in large doses, and if the patient survives this extremely serious condition, the heart muscle recovers. Fortunately, this disease has been almost eliminated by immunization.

A Picture of a Toxic Patient

A patient with a severe degree of TOXAEMIA (toxins in the blood) may be far from normal in her feelings, behaviour and appearance. She may be bright-eyed, and feel as if she is 'on fire', with a hot, dry skin, or 'in a pool of water' when she is sweating profusely. Her hair may be lifeless and bedraggled, lying matted and sticky in the nape of her neck against a saturated pillow. The pulse rate may be increased from the normal, and the respirations rapid, with foul breath. Her mouth and lips may be dry with unpleasant deposits on the teeth and gums, and although she may be unusually thirsty, everything given to her to drink is said to be tasteless.

A worried, frowning expression may indicate that she has a headache, or the light might be bothering her. She may call out, as people do in dreams, or be obsessed with one idea—perhaps that there is a man under the bed, and will even succeed in convincing her relatives that there is! On the other hand, a patient with this condition may not realize that she is in bed in a hospital ward, but thinks she is in some very strange place, and therefore try to get out of bed to find her way home. The fact that she is dressed only in a nightgown, and may be attached to a bottle of fluid, does not seem to deter her. This obvious mental confusion may be transient only, and when her efforts to run away are stopped by a nurse, the patient may realize that she is doing something unusual, but cannot help herself.

Management of the Toxic Patient. Nurses who have had no experience of patients in this condition may be concerned and distressed to find them behaving in such an unusual way. It is therefore understandable that the patient's relatives find such a situation even more puzzling. The reassuring words given by the doctor or the sister, that the patient will respond to treatment, and will be returned to them wholly recovered, may even appear to fall on deaf ears.

There is a great deal that the nurse can do to help this patient. A group of drugs, the antipyretic group, is used to reduce pyrexia. The well-known aspirin is often used. Fluids in large quantities are given frequently (totalling several litres a day), provided kidney function is satisfactory, and the object of this treatment is to dilute the circulating toxins, and thereby make them less effective. They will be excreted in the urine.

The doctor will probably order an antibiotic to be given, and give permission for tepid sponging to be carried out, but only with good nursing will the patient be restored to her normal self. With all the body's activities speeded up, many complications have to be prevented. The patient must not be allowed to lie in damp sheets and clothing, otherwise a 'chill' may develop and lower still further her resistance to disease. The skin must be washed frequently, perhaps every four hours—or sponged with water at a temperature between 24° and 26°C. (75° and 80°F.) in an effort to reduce the temperature of the body—and the bed linen and clothing changed. The hair can be combed and rearranged, and the pillows changed to provide a fresh, clean, dry area for the patient's head.

The dry mouth and cracked lips require the attention of a capable nurse, otherwise sores will develop. Hard, boiled fruit sweets may help to make the mouth a little fresher. The pressure areas must not become red and sore. Two hourly turning of the patient is necessary if the patient is lying still in bed, accompanied by inspection of the parts of the body which may be rubbing against the bedclothes.

It is customary to record the patient's temperature, pulse and respiration rates every four hours. Scanty, concentrated urine, and whether or not the patient has diarrhoea or constipation, are important observations to be reported to the sister.

It is so very satisfying to a nurse when she realizes that her nursing of an ill, toxic patient is rewarded by the patient's gradual return to normal, and she will have discovered that working with an experienced sister has taught her a greal deal. Textbooks play a part, but they can never take the place of the real patient in a living situation.

FURTHER READING
Taverner, *Physiology for Nurses*. E.U.P.

CHAPTER 23

THE NURSE AND THE ELDERLY PATIENT

When a baby is born it is quite helpless and needs a great deal of attention if it is to live. As month succeeds month and year succeeds year the child becomes less and less dependent on others, until it finally achieves independence. There is no set age for this to happen, but once independence has been gained, it is generally taken for granted. As long as the adult is healthy, both in body and mind, any sort of activity can be indulged in, with much pleasure and satisfaction.

As the years go by there is a gradual slowing down of activity, but the changes are hardly noticeable. The vigorous outdoor sports lose some of their appeal. Certain activities need more conscious effort; glasses may be needed, and a hearing aid may be necessary. Not only physical activity is affected; older people tend to dislike changes and their mental outlook becomes narrower. The 'bounce' of youth disappears and caution takes its place. Leaving work and retiring is a major step, especially for a man who has worked hard and enjoyed earning his living.

Elderly people vary greatly in their reactions to the processes of ageing. There is no definite age in years (referred to as chronological age) at which everyone can be said to be old. Some people give up all effort in their sixties, others are wonderfully active in their eighties. When a loved one dies, the ageing processes in the one left behind are hastened, and if bereavement means removal to unfamiliar surroundings as well, then deterioration is often rapid.

Characteristics of Old Age

Whatever the outlook of the individual, certain physical characteristics are inescapable. Hair loses its colour, and is white or grey; men may become very thin 'on top', or hair may disappear completely. The skin of an old person may become wrinkled and lined. There are very few who have more than a couple of odd teeth. The hearing may not be as good as it was, and they may find difficulty in seeing things clearly. Muscular movement is slower, bones become brittle and may break easily. Old people seldom require large meals as the appetite is diminished. The circulation of the blood and the pulse are slower, extremities are cold, and because there is less blood to the brain, mental processes are often affected. Sons and daughters may notice that their parents are forgetful, have got into the habit of repeating 'Wait a minute', and take much longer to think out answers to simple questions.

Unfortunately many old people are less fastidious than they used to be. Having a bath is such an effort that they neglect personal cleanliness, and fail to use deodorants. Carelessness creeps in at mealtimes too, clothing may be spotted with food, and either because of poor sight or laziness the clothes are not washed or cleaned. A number of old people present a rather neglected picture.

Elderly People in Hospital

Many hospital patients are old and nurses must realize that they may be there for many reasons. One old person may be in hospital because of a degenerative condition, e.g. arteriosclerosis—due almost entirely to the processes of ageing. Another may be suffering from an illness which could affect any age group, e.g. bronchitis. Old people are more prone to accidents, because of failing eyesight and other factors, and whereas a young person may escape with a few bruises in a fall, the old person will probably break a bone. There may be quite a large number of elderly people in the accident wards. Occasionally old people are victims of social and economic pressures, may develop deficiency diseases, like scurvy, or may be admitted to hospital purely as social problems, because there is no one for them to live with.

Elderly patients are found throughout the whole of a general hospital, with the exception of the children's and maternity wards. The nursing care is almost the same as for the other patients, but greater care must be taken to avoid complications. Frequent change of position and attention to pressure areas may prevent pressure sores. Confinement to bed is avoided as much as possible, but if the patient is not encouraged to get out of the chair, and move, the chair may be as lethal as the bed. Adequate support for the back is necessary at all times, and the old person is taught to breathe deeply, to prevent respiratory complications. The physiotherapist will visit to help in these and other exercises. Small meals should be provided and extra nourishment in the form of milk drinks with added glucose and protein given if necessary. The nurse may have to assist with personal toilet but she will find that although the old people take a little longer to become fully mobile, many make remarkable recoveries from major surgery or accidents. They cheerfully leave hospital to resume their former way of life.

Unfortunately for other patients, recovery is long delayed, or prevented by complications. It is even sadder, when an old person recovers but cannot return home because of unwilling relatives or landlord. Some may be left with a disability which handicaps their return to awkward home conditions, e.g. it might be impossible for them to cope with stairs. There are a number of old people who are transferred to geriatric units, or admitted to an Old Folks' Home, after a stay in hospital.

Elderly people suffering from degenerative diseases need treatment and care in hospital. They may recover sufficiently to return home for a time, but sooner or later, continuous care will be essential.

Finally, there is the category of the old who are social problems, suffering perhaps from malnutrition or senility. Of all the afflictions of the elderly probably senility is the saddest. These old people are confused, they do not remember where they are, become distressed because they know they cannot remember, and there seems to be little reasoning behind actions and words. They may not recognize relatives, and sometimes they are noisy and abusive, especially if anyone tries to remonstrate with them.

The Elderly in a Geriatric Unit

In a geriatric unit there are a variety of patients—some will be up and about and others in bed; some cheerful and some depressed, and a number will be senile. All of them need and deserve the highest standards of nursing care, and many nurses find that this type of work is very satisfying.

The care of these elderly citizens must be organized on three planes—physical, mental, and spiritual.

Physical Care

Each patient must be kept clean and comfortable at all times. A daily bath must be given—an ordinary general bath, a shower, or a complete wash at a hand basin—whichever is easiest for the patient. The nails must be kept short and clean. The mouth requires attention before and after meals or feeds; hair is brushed and arranged carefully, and is washed regularly. If the elderly patient is thin, or obese, the pressure areas must be relieved very frequently. The use of a hoist may be helpful in lifting patients, and when changing their positions. (See fig. 81)

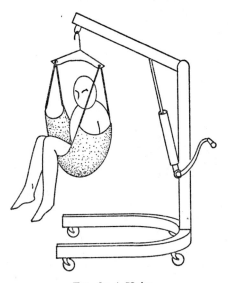

FIG. 81 A Hoist

The nurse must be particularly careful to see that the bladder and bowels are functioning properly. Old people sometimes have a diminished output of urine simply because they do not drink enough. More often they are incontinent of urine, and the nurse has then to deal with this unhappy state of affairs. Having satisfied herself that the patient is not suffering from retention with overflow, the nurse must do all that she can to keep the patient dry. Putting the patient on a commode, lavatory or bedpan, at regular short intervals will sometimes establish a habit which will empty the bladder. The use of disposable pads often saves a great amount of laundry. Wet and soiled clothes must be changed at once. Dressing the elderly in their own clothes will often encourage them to keep clean and dry—incontinence is seen much more often in patients confined to bed.

Faecal incontinence is more distressing to the patient and more unpleasant for the nurse. It may be due to an overful bowel and emptying the colon with suppositories or an enema may cure the condition. Nurses should observe whether any particular food leads to diarrhoea and then incontinence. Omission of that food may cure the incontinence.

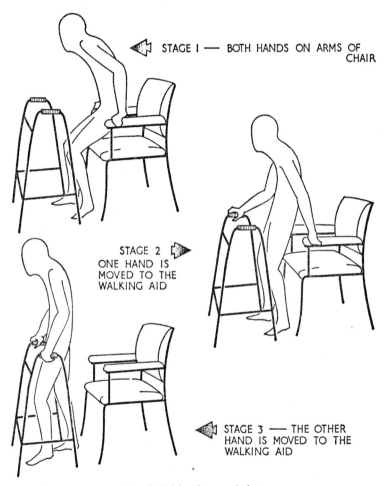

STAGE I — BOTH HANDS ON ARMS OF CHAIR

STAGE 2 ONE HAND IS MOVED TO THE WALKING AID

STAGE 3 — THE OTHER HAND IS MOVED TO THE WALKING AID

Fig. 82 Rising from a chair

It is never helpful to reproach patients who have lost control but a word of praise on dry days is very encouraging.

The diet must not be overlooked. Food should be appetizing, of the correct Calorie value and contain all the essential foodstuffs, including vitamins and minerals. Sometimes an inadequate diet is taken because the old person has either lost his dentures or simply refuses to wear them. The ingenuity of the nurse is challenged, as she has to find ways of providing the necessary nourishment. Milk is very useful—it is not exclusively for the young.

Old people need not be dressed in drab and shapeless garments, whether in or out of bed, and they should wear their own clothing as much as possible. Clothing which is easily washed and drips dry is helpful—nylon, brushed nylon, tricel, and in particular turkish towelling dressing-gowns, are all good.

As these patients are up and dressed, unless there is a definite reason for them not to be, a garden attached to a day room provides a refreshing change of environment, and is conducive to sleeping better. Exercise is essential, and sitting in a chair for hours on end is just about as harmful as staying in bed. The physiotherapist must teach the patient the skilled technique of rising from a chair.

Warmth is also essential. Most elderly people feel the cold, and if a building is cold they will tend to sit near to the fire and be reluctant to move. Central heating is ideal. An even temperature does not hinder movement. Bathroom and lavatories too should be warm, otherwise the patient will try to avoid using them and skimp washing.

A small glass of whisky or brandy as a nightcap, especially if the patient has always had one, saves much confusion and deterioration which often follows the giving of sedatives, e.g. barbiturates.

Mental and Spiritual Care

Every effort should be made to keep the elderly interested and active. Visits from families and friends should be encouraged by all day open visiting, and whenever possible outings should be arranged for half-days, days, weekends or even holidays. Some elderly people have no relations and have outlived their friends, so local voluntary organizations, Red Cross, and St. John's can often help. Radio and television programmes are interesting and occupational therapists can often find small pieces of work to provide mental stimulus.

Many elderly patients are taken to church services, and during the week the hospital chaplains and outside ministers keep in touch and get to know the patients very well.

Above all, the old need courtesy, kindness and consideration. Calling them 'gran' and 'dad', for instance, is not appreciated and may be justifiably resented.

It is necessary sometimes for hospital authorities to make arrangements to admit geriatric patients for 2 or 3 weeks once or twice a year, so that the relatives who care for them at home, may go away for a holiday.

Prevention of Disease

Although it is inevitable that some old people will need institutional care, every effort should be made to keep them independent as long as possible. Sometimes support in the home is all that is required and this may be organized by the Health Visitor. Home helps, the meals-on-wheels service, and laundry services, will relieve the burden of domestic chores. Home visits are made by many voluntary organizations—perhaps for purely social reasons, or to help with the shopping, give a bath—write a letter—or read to the old person. In every case contact with others makes old people feel that they matter to someone.

From the practical point of view regular visiting does ensure that the elderly, if they do meet with an accident in the home, are not left indefinitely before someone finds them. Street visiting has been organized by some churches, so there is constant contact between the churchgoers, the place of worship, and the shut-in old person.

Within the last few years some pioneers have started clinics and day hospitals for old people, for the practice of preventive medicine. Medical examinations reveal early signs of disease and degeneration; dieticians ensure that an adequate amount of the right foods are being eaten, and a chiropody service treats corns and ingrowing toenails that may be preventing ambulation.

A small amount of care and supervision of health may keep old people active and happy in their own homes, and prevent the occurrence of many major diseases.

FURTHER READING

Adams & McIlwraith, *Geriatric Nursing: A study of the Work of Geriatric Ward Staff.* Oxford University Press.

Agate, *The Practice of Geriatrics.* Heinemann.

Agate, (1st October 1966) *Accidents to Old People in Their Homes.* British Medical Journal.

Exton-Smith, Norton and McLaren, *An Investigation of Geriatric Nursing Problems in Hospital.* National Corporation for the Care of Old People.

Irvine, R. *et al. The Older Patient.* E.U.P.

Rudd, *Nursing of the Elderly Sick.* Faber and Faber.

Shaw, *Old People in Homes.* Faber and Faber.

Wallis, Gwynneth, *Guide to Activities for Older People.* Elek Books.

Westropp & Williams, *Health and Happiness in Old Age.* Methuen.

Health for Old Age. Consumer Association.

CHAPTER 24

THE NURSE AND THE DYING PATIENT

It is a paradox that some people conceal from their children the facts about the two most basic things in the world—birth and death. Most parents and many teachers do make an attempt to tell children something about the former. The latter, the only certainty in nature, is often ignored. The majority of young people who enter a training school do so with little or no idea of what death entails. Most nurses do not think very much about this subject until just before their training starts, and they rarely ask about it. Everyone is apprehensive about the unknown, so most nurses are rather frightened at the prospect of being with someone when they die. In actual fact, death is not a frightening process; it is a sad one, and the grief of relatives may be hard to bear, but fear is not often present. Death comes in many ways, sometimes suddenly, and sometimes so peacefully that it is almost impossible to perceive the moment of dying.

The Nurse's Reaction
The problems created by this situation are very real ones for the nurse. Her reactions depend on her personality and past experiences. Death is an ever-present reality in nursing practice. It is a time of crisis for the patient, the relatives, and the doctors and nurses who attend the patient. Some doctors and nurses tend to 'deny' the fact of death, and may adopt the traditional detached professional attitude, in order to cope with, or escape from, the situation.

Difficulties in dealing with a dying patient tend to spring from personal and emotional factors, from the nurse's own anxieties, rather than from any problem concerned with the actual practical nursing care of the patient. The problems, although personal and complex, can sometimes be thought about and borne more easily if opportunities have been provided early on in the nurse training course for discussion with senior nurses, doctors and chaplains.

Some nurses may have had extremely painful experiences of

loss through death, and are therefore unusually sensitive. Others find that the death of a patient in a certain age group causes great stress; the death of a child, or of a patient in the same age group as the nurse. The nurse's emotional reaction may be complex. She may feel pity, despair, sorrow or fear. She may worry because she is emotionally affected, or she may worry because she is not. She may find, to her own disquiet, that the strongest emotion is of being glad to be alive, and that she is trying to shut out her feelings about the patient by avoiding his bedside. She may worry lest he should ask her questions which she cannot answer, such as 'Have I got cancer?' 'Am I ever going to go home?' There are no easy answers to these questions, and whilst she is in a junior capacity, the responsibility of giving direct answers does not rest with her. The nurse follows the sister's instructions.

The Patient's Attitude

The attitude of patients to death vary greatly. Whether or not the patient should be told he is dying is one of the most controversial points in medicine. Nurses may be very concerned about the assumption so often made by people that a patient does not know about his illness. Patients commonly know far more about their illnesses, even approaching death, than many people give them credit for. Many patients want to be told the truth, and are often grateful for the opportunity of talking frankly about their feelings.

The patient may be the first to talk about his condition, and help himself by finding, as it were, his own solution, or partial solution, to his problems. If he asks questions like 'Do you think I am going to get better?' they are best answered by counter-questions, such as 'Well, what do you think? Are you feeling any better?' If patients do ask straight out, and if they have been told the truth by the doctor, for a short time there is an obvious emotional upset, but after this there is far greater mental peace. There is no doubt that those who suffer, almost always find the strength with which to carry the burden. (Exceptions should be made with extremely nervous people, but even they should not be put off with 'stories' or deliberate lies.) In some situations it seems that the unwillingness to tell a patient is because the person upon whose shoulders this responsibility should fall, is reluctant to perform an unpleasant task.

Every nurse is bound to have her own views on whether the patient should be told that chances of recovery are very slight, and at some time she will be involved in the implementation of decisions made by doctors and sisters. It is hard to justify, on any grounds, the string of 'stories' invented, and the false hopes which are sometimes aroused, in an attempt to preserve the patient's peace of mind. The patient quickly becomes suspicious, and deceitful practices could cause him much more mental agony than the sober truth.

Some patients never voice their feelings, but it is obvious they know they are going to die and they are not afraid. They know the subject of death is a distressing one, and they seem to deliberately avoid mentioning it, so that their loved ones do not have the sadness of discussing it. Very old patients appear to welcome death. Life has run its course, and when the powers of the body can no longer fulfil the demands of the mind, the person often finds life a burden they willingly relinquish. Some old people lose much of their mental awareness and to these death is a quiet ending to a sad chapter of their lives.

When patients know their true condition, they should receive careful attention. A great deal can be done to relieve physical pain and discomfort, but the emotional and spiritual needs of the patients should not be forgotten, and every effort should be made to help them.

The Patient's Emotional and Spiritual Needs

It is not within the scope of any textbook to even outline a plan of care which would meet the emotional and spiritual needs of every dying patient. Comfort and care must be given to each individual according to his requirements, and can only be given by those who are prepared to listen and to try to understand and help. The nurse is often nearest to the patient, and therefore able to help him most. She has a primary role to play. Listening to what he has to say with sympathy and compassion will be the most important aspect of her care. Nursing 'busy-ness' and efficiency may prevent conversation, and may result in a patient dying in what has been called a state of 'demoralised vegetation', without dignity and in a turmoil.

It is necessary for nurses to co-operate with hospital chaplains and ministers of all faiths in helping to meet the spiritual needs of the patient. Every man has a soul, and during a terminal illness he probably thinks more about its welfare than at any other time. Those whose faith has sustained them in life turn to it for support in death. Those without faith may be helped to find it in their hour of need. A hospital chaplain will visit the patient, and visits may also be paid by the priest or minister from the patient's own church. Many Christians will wish to receive Holy Communion. Roman Catholic patients will, in addition, receive a special Sacrament before death, and nurses should make sure that the priest has been notified of any deterioration in the patient's condition.

Nurse's Attitude Towards the Relatives

The doctor will give all the information he can to the relatives, but the nurse may have to explain again some of his statements. In no way should she add to the information already given. Having to deal with relatives is an additional responsibility for the nurse, but her kindness and consideration go a long way towards alleviating their distress. They should not be allowed to gather round the bed of the patient, as this may deprive him of necessary air. It is not within the nurse's province to turn relatives away, but the relatives should arrange their own visiting order—generally only two at the bedside at one time. They may even assist the nurse with some of the nursing duties. Helping to change the patient's position, or wiping his face, may help them a little in their grief.

If the patient is restless, or shows that he may be in pain, an explanation should be given to the relatives. The nurse can remind them that medications to prevent pain and discomfort are being given, and that these reactions are not necessarily signs of physical distress. Relatives who have not seen the patient in the late stages of his illness might be overwhelmed at the change in him. They must be warned by the nurse, before they see the patient, and asked not to give way to an uncontrolled display of grief. Most hospitals have visitors' rooms where relatives may stay, and where meals may be served to them.

P

The Patient at Home

If the course of the terminal illness is going to be of some length, patients are often much happier in their own homes. In familiar surroundings, cared for by their own relatives, they can enjoy their last weeks. Before sending the patient home, however, sister and the doctor will have assured themselves that conditions are suitable. Support must be given to relatives by the district nurse if necessary. A home help may go to the house for a few hours each day and some local authorities have a night visiting organization which may be very valuable. These patients will probably return to hospital eventually and some patients may be too ill even to contemplate going home in the first place.

Care of the Dying Patient

The nursing care of these patients is devoted to one end—keeping them comfortable in every way. This includes the prevention of any complication which would add to their distress. Such things as a pressure sore, a dirty mouth, a distended bladder or a rectum full of hard faeces are all discomforts which no patient properly nursed should ever have; they are unforgivable in a dying patient. Careful and unhurried attention must be given, and the ward routine adapted to suit the patient, not the other way round. The patient is nursed in the position of the greatest comfort, and turned when necessary. As he becomes weaker he may slide down in the bed and sometimes raising the foot of it will keep him in an easier position without disturbing him to lift him up so often. He will appreciate extra support for his head with a small pillow.

It is easy for such a patient to become dehydrated and nurse should see that the patient drinks at least two litres (three pints) each day. Even someone near the end of his life can still enjoy a favourite food and this should be provided if at all possible. The appearance of the patient is important. Nurses take pride in seeing that bed linen is spotless and that pyjamas and nightdresses are clean. Men must be shaved and their hair kept tidy, being cut if necessary. Women should have their hair arranged in an attractive style, and if they want to wear lipstick and nail varnish this should be put on with care. Sometimes the patient may have a wound with an offensive discharge. Dressings must be changed frequently and a deodorant spray may be used. At this time the patient feels more alone than ever before and may find a bell a comfort to him. He will not wish to be disturbed constantly by the nurse asking questions, but will appreciate it if she comes to his bedside at regular intervals, even though he may not want to speak to her.

The Use of Drugs

Many people fear death because they feel it will be painful. In actual fact very few diseases cause pain and in any event there is no reason why the patient should suffer. There are many drugs which relieve pain, and they should be used intelligently and freely in a terminal illness. The aim is to prevent pain being felt, rather than 'killing' the pain when it has reached a peak. Doctors often vary the type and timing of analgesics they give the patient. This is done to find the drug which suits the patient best and also because a change of drug sometimes makes the patient feel better. For severe pain opium, or one of its derivatives, is the best analgesic of all. Morphia or heroin relieve pain and promote sleep and have no equal. The nurse may be distressed and alarmed to find that the dosage of analgesic drugs may be very large indeed. In effect, of course, the patient has become addicted to the drug, and the large doses are necessary for it to have its normal effect on him. As there is no chance of his recovery there is no reason for withholding the drugs. Because of this addiction, however, they are not prescribed in the earlier stages of the illness. They are held in reserve until the right moment has come to use them.

Signs of Approaching Death

Each day sees a deterioration in the patient's condition. The pulse weakens, the patient finds it more difficult to move, and in many cases he loses full consciousness of his surroundings. Respirations tend to become noisier and shallower. The noise, which is very distressing to the relatives, can often be minimised by a change of position. Noisy respirations usually occur when the patient is lying flat on his back. Raising the head and shoulders on to two or three pillows, or turning the patient on to one side often reduces the noise considerably. The skin feels cold to the touch and is sometimes covered with perspiration.

P*

There is extreme pallor of the face and there may be cyanosis round the lips. The patient does not appear to be able to see properly and he rarely speaks coherently. He may, however, be able to hear and this should not be forgotten when nurses or relatives are talking. Whispering does not help the patient and it may only disturb him more. Normal tones in conversation should be used. If the patient has relatives they will usually be with him at this stage so that the patient is rarely left alone. The mere physical presence of someone else at the bedside may be a comfort, although often for a few hours before death the patient is totally unaware of his surroundings. The actual moment of death occurs when the heart stops beating and respirations cease. When this happens relatives often prefer to be left alone for a few moments, then they are accompanied to the waiting room or office. They are seen here by sister or her deputy and allowed to wait a short time before going home. No details of certificates, clothing or other property are discussed; the relatives go home and arrangements are made for one member of the family to return the next day to deal with all the official business. If possible the patient's relatives should never return home alone, and a friend or neighbour may be contacted who will make sure that they are all right.

Although the care of the patient is the nurse's undisputed work, her compassion must extend to the relatives if it is felt that they too are in need of support. Hospital chaplains will readily help by talking with relatives, and the hospital communications system generally provides for chaplains to be easily and quickly called to wards and departments.

Care of the Body After Death

Following instructions from sister, the nurse who was with the patient removes the pillows except one, and gently straightens the body. There is an exception to this in the case of Orthodox Jews who must be attended by members of their own faith. If the lower jaw sags open it should be supported and the eyes closed, then the face is covered and the body is left.

Hospitals now vary in their practices. In some hospitals the nurses are instructed to straight away remove any tubes attached to the patient, replace dentures, and apply clean dressings. A large pad is placed over the genitalia and if necessary clean night clothes are placed on the patient. A written note is made on the identification card of any jewellery left on the patient. The bottom sheet, if clean, is used to wrap around the patient, and he is taken from the ward as soon as possible.

In other hospitals, about an hour after death, two nurses attend to the last offices. Any wounds have a clean dressing applied, kept in position by occlusive strapping. Pressure over the lower abdomen will empty the bladder into a receiver placed between the thighs. The body should then be washed and clothed in a shroud. The nails should be cleaned and the hair arranged tidily. All jewellery is removed, although sometimes relatives prefer to leave a wedding ring on the finger. A card of identification is attached and then the body is wrapped in a special sheet.

Porters now bring a special trolley to the ward and remove the body to the mortuary. Curtains should be drawn round the beds so that other patients do not see this. They are, of course, aware of what is happening but they can be spared the actual sight of the body being removed. In many hospitals a nurse accompanies the porters to the mortuary entrance.

In the ward the bedclothes are sent to the laundry and the mattress and pillows are removed. They may be autoclaved or left out in the air and sunshine before being used again. The contents of the locker are carefully checked and listed, then sent to the hospital office; relatives collect them from there.

Effect on Other Patients

Nurses must remember that all the patients in the ward are profoundly affected by the death of one of their number. Although they do not talk about the situation they have all taken note of the drawn curtains and the extra screen. They have watched the relatives being escorted to and from the bedside, and they have observed the facial expressions and manner of all those who have passed in and out of the screens. They have heard a great deal of what has passed between the nurses, the patient and his relatives, and have noted the behaviour of those who have cared for the patient. It is important that the nurse's manner should be calm and dignified at all times so that the other patients and the relatives may draw strength from her.

Some people react to death in a hysterical and inappropriate way and this, although it may only be a manifestation of immature behaviour, could easily be misunderstood and cause great distress to others.

Family Responsibilities

In straightforward cases the relatives are told to visit the hospital the next day and they are then given the death certificate. This gives the time and cause of death and is signed by the doctor. The relatives have then to go to the Registrar to register the death, and once that is done the undertaker can remove the body.

In some cases the doctor may wish to examine the body from the point of view of interest. He has to obtain permission from the relatives to do this, and they may refuse if they so wish. On the other hand sometimes the cause of death is unknown, or the patient dies in rather suspicious circumstances. The doctor cannot then sign the death certificate and it is his duty to inform the coroner of the circumstances. If the coroner feels that a post mortem examination is necessary, the relatives are notified but they cannot, in this instance, withhold their permission.

Making a Will

The making of a will is the responsibility of the patient, his legal advisers, and even of his family. If the nurse is asked to witness a will, or write anything down, she must ascertain from the sister in charge of the ward the exact requirements of the hospital in such a matter, before involving herself, and the hospital. Nurses are not themselves concerned with these administrative details, but they should be aware of them in case they are asked about them by relatives.

Help for Nurses

Nurses do get attached to their patients and they feel upset and sad when those patients die. This is a very natural feeling, and it would be a very poor nurse who did not feel upset at the loss of someone she had grown to know. She may find that a talk with the hospital chaplain or her priest may be helpful at this time if she is upset and confused by the fact of death.

There is always some compensation in feeling that the patient received every attention and all possible care during his last illness. No good nurse ever loses an opportunity to demonstrate that whatever happens she 'comforts always.'

FURTHER READING

Bird, B., *Talking with Patients*. Lippincott.

Hinton, John, *Dying*. Penguin

Kübler-Ross, E., *On Death and Dying*. Tavistock.

Saunders, C., *Care of the Dying*. Nursing Times Reprint.

Blackwell and Worcester, A., *The Care of the Aged, the Dying and the Dead*. Oxford.

Murray Parkes, Colin, *Bereavement*, Tavistock.

CHAPTER 25

THE PATIENT'S RETURN HOME

At last the day comes when the patient is ready to return home. All arrangements have been made, the doctor will have talked to the patient and his wife at times during the preceding weeks and discussed with them any problems they may have concerning the condition of the patient, and possible changes in his future life. The medical social worker will have seen the patient and given any advice necessary about his future and his finances. Because the patient is moving from one part of the health service to another (from the hospital service to the general practitioner and community service) much liaison is necessary so that the patient shall suffer no inconvenience by the move. A letter will have been sent to the patient's general practitioner explaining what treatment the patient has had and is now having. If home nursing will be needed, the home nurse will be notified. In many cases the nursing officer from the local authority service visits the hospital regularly and will therefore know of the patients discharge, otherwise the home nurse is telephoned.

Leaving the Ward

Sister has made sure that any medicines or dressings the patient is taking home with him have been fetched from the Pharmacy and that his valuables have been fetched from the safe. She has also given him his last intermediate certificate for sickness benefit, and explained that any further intermediate certificates and the final certificate will all be obtained from his own doctor. A 'follow-up' appointment has been made in the Out Patient Department and the patient has his appointment card. Finally his wife comes with his clothes and sister will take this opportunity to have a word with her whilst nurse is helping the patient to dress. Then when all the accumulation of belongings in the locker have been safely packed, and the pyjamas which nurse kindly washed have been remembered and rescued from the bathroom, the patient, looking strangely different in his own clothes, makes his farewell tour of his friends. At last, with nurse going down to see them to the taxi, the patient and his wife leave the hospital.

Transfer to Convalescent Home

However, not all discharges follow this simple pattern. There are some patients whose home circumstances are not suitable for them during the time which must elapse before they are fit to return to work. There are some who are unlikely to be able to resist the temptation to do too much if they return home immediately. For these patients a stay at a convalescent home is ideal. Arranging for this is one of the duties of the medical social worker, and not always an easy one. Vacancies do not always occur when the patient is ready for discharge. Some homes are unable to accept patients having special diets, others have no lifts so all their patients must be able to climb stairs. Patients sometimes find at the last minute that they cannot stand the thought of longer separation from their children and cancel the plans which have been made for them. Usually, however, patients enjoy their time in a convalescent home and return home rested.

Special Problems

Real problems arise when the patient on his discharge must, either temporarily or permanently, alter his way of life. An example of such adaptation is the patient with a colostomy. (A colostomy is an opening from the bowel on to the abdominal wall so that the patient discharges faeces through this opening). Preparation for his discharge has, of course, started long before he actually leaves the hospital. The explanation and acceptance of a colostomy start before operation. Afterwards the nurse teaches the patient to care for his colostomy himself, but even when he has learnt this in hospital, he must be able to adapt to home conditions. In hospital there is a bathroom, hot water, cotton wool, gauze and a good supply of clean linen; boxes of disposable colostomy bags appear in the cupboard on stores day, and a nurse is always available to lend a hand if required. At home the patient will want to know such things as 'where will I be able to get a colostomy bag in the High Street? Which is the cheaper, cotton wool or cellulose wadding?' Several people can help here, but the most useful is a former patient with a colostomy. Although hospitals supply special leaflets about how to care for a colostomy, and special diet sheets are discussed with the patient and his wife, only someone *with* a colostomy can advise with real sincerity on practical points which worry the patient and his wife. (Groups of ex-patients with other conditions besides colostomies are now in existence, for example, The Swallow Club whose members have all had a laryngectomy).

Mental Adjustments

Another way in which former patients can help is in reassuring the patients about the way they will feel. Only someone who has had such a condition can fully understand the feelings of bitterness and resentment the patient has. Whilst he was in hospital he was ill and frightened and grateful for all that was done for him, once he has returned home he has more time to turn over and over in his mind that unanswerable question, 'Why did it have to happen to me?' He stops being thankful for being alive and remembers only the burden of being disabled. He also needs reassurance about his fitness, he should be warned of the long time there may be between being told he is better and feeling well in himself. A patient who is well enough for discharge may not FEEL really well for weeks or even months afterwards. At length the patient, who has been attended at home by both his doctor and the district nurse is able to dispense with their support (except for regular visits for prescriptions) and gradually adapt himself to his new life. In fact, once the colostomy has been accepted it need not alter the patient's way of life at all. Thousands of people, doctors, nurses, actors and shopkeepers manage their colostomies without anyone but their families being aware that they have one.

Change of Occupation

There are, however, other conditions which may necessitate a complete change in the patient's manner of living. Some people, it is true, manage to continue with disabilities that would daunt others, but not all pilots can continue to fly after the loss of both legs, nor all composers continue to write music after they have lost their hearing. Many people have to face the fact that they must change their job following accident or illness. This is never easy. Really severe disabilities such as blindness require a long period of training both for normal living and another job, usually in a residential centre. Other patients with disabilities are dealt with by the disablement resettlement

officers attached to every local authority who arrange for
patients to go to retraining workshops in various parts of
the country. The real difficulty lies in equating what the
patient wants to do with what he is able to do. A young
woman who has had to give up nursing because of sensitivity
to drugs may have set her heart on being a nurse since she
was a little girl, and it may take time for her to get used to
the idea of another job.

Rehabilitation

Sometimes a disability is not sufficiently serious to prevent a
patient returning to his former work, but he needs some time
before he is able to regain his old skill. Many firms have special
rehabilitation workshops for such workers. Here the patient
works at such tasks and for such hours as the doctor in charge
thinks suitable, but takes back a full wage packet at the end of
the week. The machine at which he works has been specially
adapted for his particular disability. Every handle he moves
or screw he turns helps to strengthen a weak muscle or loosen
a stiff joint, yet the articles he produces are all being made use
of in the factory. A period in such a workshop makes the transi-
tion back to full work much easier both mentally and physically.
The patient does not have to spend a long demoralizing period
at home feeling both useless and in the way, living on his sickness
benefit. In certain instances the patient will never be able to
work at the pace required in a modern factory, but he may be
found a place in a 'sheltered workshop' such as a Remploy
factory, where special conditions exist for the employees.

Home Care

Finally there is the patient whose condition has been only
partially relieved by his stay in hospital and who may never
return to work. The elderly patient who has had a stroke, or the
patient whose heart failure is not completely controlled by
digitalis, for example, may require varying amounts of home care
for many years. A health visitor or home nurse is usually asked
to visit the home before the patient's discharge and report on its
suitability. If he cannot walk upstairs she must see whether it
would prove possible for him to live downstairs. If he is heavy
and bedridden she must note whether there is a chance of a hoist

being installed. If the patient is incontinent she must help the family to get in touch with the laundry service run by the local authority. If the patient is going to require attention during the night she must see whether it would be possible to make use of the night sitter service. If there are nursing duties which the family cannot undertake, such as the giving of certain injections, the district nurse will have to be called upon. A family undertaking the care of such a patient, however willing they are, will require a great deal of help and support.

Institutional Care

In certain instances it proves impossible for the family to have the patient home, and in this case it is usual to transfer him to another institution. This may be a hospital for the chronically ill, an old peoples' home or a nursing home. In the past the most important thing about the transfer of such a patient seemed to be his physical state. The nurses in the hospital transferring the patient made sure that his skin was clean, his mouth fresh, his toe-nails immaculate and his scalp free from lice. Now it is realized that though these points are doubtless important, the mental state of the patient should also be taken into account. He should be warned and prepared for the impending transfer in plenty of time to let him become accustomed to the idea. His relatives should be consulted, and arrangements made for them to go with him in the ambulance if possible. There is very little provision under the health service for homes for the young, chronically sick person; all too often he is placed with elderly patients. This gap has to a certain extent been filled by the homes run by the Cheshire Foundation, where young adults are accepted and are free to live in a more hopeful atmosphere, but there are still not nearly enough vacancies.

In the course of her training a nurse meets many patients. If she has nursed them through a long or dangerous illness she will have become very attached to them. Whilst patients are very ill the burden of making decisions is taken from them and they are treated like children. The first duty of the nurse as the patient recovers is to remember that he is not a child and encourage him to take control of his affairs again and prepare for his eventual discharge. All nurses soon realize that though the hospital is very important to *them*, it is not, nor should it be, the centre of the patient's existence. To the patient, his home is the centre of his life, hospital is only an episode, albeit one he may remember with gratitude. The nurse's reward comes later when faintly familiar strangers greet her cheerfully in the street with 'Hello nurse, remember me?'

FURTHER READING

Disabilities. The Lancet.

Blunden, *I Chose to Live*. Hurst & Blackett.

Davies, Meredith, *Preventive Medicine for Nurses and Social Workers*. E.U.P.

Ritchie, *Stroke*. Faber.

INDEX